20 Natural Ways
to Reduce the Risk of
Prostate Cancer

Also by James Scala, Ph.D.:

Arthritis: Diet Against It
The High Blood Pressure Relief Diet
If You Can't/Won't Stop Smoking
Making the Vitamin Connection
The New Arthritis Relief Diet
The New Eating Right for a Bad Gut
Prescription for Longevity
25 Natural Ways to Manage Stress and Avoid Burnout
25 Natural Ways to Relieve Irritable Bowel Syndrome

20 Natural Ways to Reduce the Risk of Prostate Cancer

A Mind-Body Approach to Well-Being

James Scala, Ph.D.

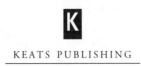

KEATS PUBLISHING

Scala, James, 1934–
　　20 natural ways to reduce the risk of prostate cancer : a mind-body approach to health and well-being / James Scala.
　　　　p.　　cm.
　　Includes index.
　　ISBN 0-658-00703-3
　　　1. Prostate—Cancer—Prevention.　　2. Prostate—Cancer—Diet therapy.
　　3. Dietary supplements.　　I. Title: Twenty natural ways to reduce the risk of prostate cancer.　　II. Title.
RC280.P7 S29　　2001
616.9′463—dc21　　　　　　　　　　　　　　　　　　　　　　　　00-066000
Published by Keats Publishing
A division of NTC/Contemporary Publishing Group, Inc.
4255 West Touhy Avenue, Lincolnwood, Illinois 60712, U.S.A.

Design by Wendy Staroba Loreen
Cover design by Mike Stromberg/The Great American Art Co.

Printed in the United States of America
International Standard Book Number: 0-658-00703-3
1 2 3 4 5 6 7 8 9 0　DOH/DOH　0 9 8 7 6 5 4 3 2 1

Contents

Introduction

You've probably heard it said, "Live long enough and you'll get prostate cancer." This simply repeats what medical research has confirmed over and over. According to the experts, prostate cancer is inevitable for every man, and your best bet is to delay its onset far enough into the future that you've simply died at a happy, comfortable, old age long before it strikes.

Delaying the onset of something scientists say is inevitable is a matter of maximizing probabilities. No person can tell you how to avoid prostate cancer with 100 percent certainty, unless that person were to suggest you have your prostate removed entirely. Specialists can tell you, however, how to improve your chances of not getting it in your lifetime—that is, how to deal with its probability realistically and intelligently.

This is not a new concept; in fact, you already deal with probabilities in some way or another every day. If you drive a car often, you will probably be involved in an accident at some point, even if you are the most cautious driver in the world. So, with that probability in mind, it makes sense to wear your seat belt and have airbags in your car. Then, when some careless driver smashes into you, your chances of coming out unscathed are vastly improved.

This is a simple, everyday example of how we use probabilities to maintain good health and avoid illness. This book's objective is to show you the steps you can take to avoid prostate cancer in your lifetime. You'll see that it is amazingly simple.

UNDERSTANDING PROSTATE CANCER

Preventing prostate cancer requires a working knowledge of how it starts, why it grows, and how it spreads. Armed with those concepts, the preventive steps will follow quite logically.

What Is Cancer?

Cancer is cell growth run amok! All cells in your body—there are about 13 trillion of them—reproduce regularly. Each tissue has its own special rate of reproduction; for example, by the time you finish this paragraph, your body will have made about 100,000 new red blood cells and discarded the remnants of the 100,000 that got old, wore out, and died. Cell reproduction is a very orderly and beautiful process that goes on throughout life. We know this process eventually ends, of course, because just as a single cell ages and dies, we, as a collective of cells, seem to share the same fate.

Sometimes a cell changes and its reproduction is no longer orderly nor true to the original. The cells produced are not normal cells; they've changed. The orderly rate of reproduction, say, every seven weeks, might be much more rapid, or just a little more rapid. As they reproduce, the new, abnormal cells begin to outnumber the normal cells, so the clump of abnormal cells keeps getting larger and eventually takes over the entire gland if not stopped. That's cancer!

Sometimes a few cells—it only takes one—from this cancerous growth break loose, find their way into a blood or lymphatic vessel, get carried along with either blood or lymph fluid, and land somewhere else in the body. If the cell or cells that break loose land where conditions are favorable, they resume their rapid reproduction, and a new cancer gets started. The cancer has now spread and may be widely dispersed throughout the body. Alternatively, the cancer may stay put. As the tumor goes undetected and gets larger, however, it might reach the membrane that encloses the gland or organ it began in, grow right through it, and become attached to surrounding tissue. Again, the cancer has spread, but it is still somewhat confined.

Because a prostate cancer cell is different and reproduces differently from other prostate cells, it follows that something in its genetic makeup has changed. How?

If scientists knew exactly and completely why a prostate cell becomes a prostate cancer cell, they could make prostate cancer—and any other cancer—disappear. There is still much for research to accomplish, but we have a good working knowledge of how the transition from a normal cell to a cancer cell takes place; we can do a lot to prevent this transition.

The transition of a cell from normal to cancerous encompasses several phases. First, a normal cell becomes *somewhat* different; it's not normal, but it is not yet a cancer cell either. Scientists refer to it as a *dysplastic cell,* which simply means it's displaced from normal and in a sort of intermediate stage. A clump of cells in this dysplastic phase can go back to being normal.

Once the cells go through the dysplastic phase and make the final transition, they become cancer cells. At that point, cancer has started to grow and the cells are forever different. They reproduce more rapidly than surrounding tissue, can develop their own blood supply, start spreading, and, if not stopped, can destroy any tissue or organ in which they arise.

Some event must change the genetic information inside the cell that causes it to become dysplastic. Whatever initiates this event is called the *initiator.* Since the transition is far more complex, however, it follows that some conditions favor the action of initiators, and other conditions then promote the transition from dysplasia to cancer. These latter conditions are lumped under the term *promoters.* Think of the initiators as the "hit men" of this criminal activity we call cancer. Think of the promoters as the environment that gives the hit men a place to live and practice their deadly deed, making the cell cancerous. Our objective is to avoid initiators and to eliminate promoters as much as is humanly and practically possible.

Initiators

Initiators cover a wide range; some can be avoided and some can't. For example, cosmic rays are initiators; they are subatomic particles that originate at the center of our galaxy, about 50,000 light-years away, and if one strikes a cell at just the right time and place, it will start the cancer process. To avoid cosmic rays, you would literally have to live in a lead mine—a rather impractical idea!

Other initiators seem quite obvious. Studies conducted over many years have helped us understand them more clearly. Some of these initiators follow:

- Chemicals that cause cancer in animal testing. About half of the 1,500 new chemicals introduced annually are tested for their ability to cause cancer in animal studies. Those tested are ones that are most likely to enter the environment.
- Numerous studies comparing people show that those who work with chemicals have a much higher cancer rate than matched controls working for the same companies in a different capacity, say, accounting.
- Men who work with automotive chemicals, such as solvents, lubricating fluids, and similar substances, are much more likely to get male breast cancer.
- Childhood cancer is most likely to develop in children whose parent (or parents) work with chemicals, such as solvents and cleaning fluids. That implies that the initiators can affect one person (a child) and not others (the parent).
- Smoking and tobacco use. Just about every type of cancer, including prostate, is higher in people who smoke. Every

puff of tobacco smoke or drop of juice from chewing tobacco contains carcinogens (initiators).

- Radiation (including the cosmic rays discussed above).
- Chlorinated pesticides. These pesticides are generally designed to interfere with the hormonal systems of insects. Women and men who are exposed consistently to them are more likely to develop breast cancer.
- Oxidizing agents. Whenever we breathe in exhaust fumes, expose ourselves to ultraviolet radiation or some solvents, or physically exert ourselves, we establish favorable conditions for oxidizing agents, which cause production of free radicals. A free radical is short-lived (0.001 second or less) and can cause genetic damage.

As you can see, initiators are all around. Suppose you spill a little gasoline on your hand while filling your tank and stand in the bright sunlight at the gas station by the freeway breathing exhaust fumes. Then you get back into your car and continue on your trip while munching on an apple that was treated with pesticides while growing and possibly sprayed with a substance to make it shiny. In just this short amount of time, a number of possible initiators emerge.

You cannot avoid all initiators. You can take many steps, however, to minimize their entry into your body. For example, wash your hands after pumping the gas, wash the apple, and wear a hat. In chapter 1, we'll explore nature's own defense system to prevent the action of these initiators. Now let's turn our attention to the promoters.

Promoters

Thanks to the unrelenting work of modern medical epidemiologists, cancer promotion is well understood. In general, we do it to ourselves! Some of these promoters follow:

- High-fat diet. The greater the dietary calorie percentage of saturated fat (generally animal fat), the higher the rate of cancer.

- Red meat (generally beef) consumption. The more frequently people eat meat, the more likely they are to develop cancer. For example, the colon cancer rate in people who eat beef five times weekly is 3.5 times greater than for those who eat it once a month; the rate is similar for prostate cancer.
- Low-fiber diet. In general, people whose diet is low in fiber do not eat enough cereals, grains, fruits, and vegetables. The cancer rates in these people are higher. Similarly, people who are chronically constipated (due to low fiber intake) have higher cancer rates.
- Poor vegetable and fruit habits. People who avoid fruits and vegetables or simply don't bother to eat them are more likely to develop cancer, including prostate cancer.
- Poor fitness. Excessive weight and lack of exercise increase the risk of most cancers, including prostate cancer.
- High testosterone levels and testosterone metabolites. Cancers of the prostate start in an environment in which testosterone helps them grow. Men often take substances to increase testosterone.
- Family history of prostate cancer. In chapter 1, we'll discuss nature's safeguards against cancer. It's possible that an inborn genetic predisposition can make a man more likely to get prostate cancer.

There are many things we can do to reduce prostate cancer risk. In fact, the above information illustrates that we have the ability to prevent and avoid most cancer promoters or at least reduce our risk to an absolute minimum.

When you consider the number of cancer initiators and promoters we face every day, it's amazing that life expectancy is presently almost eighty years. Life has been developing on Earth for about four billion years and man has been here for about three million years; many of these initiators and promoters have been around for at least that long. Shouldn't we expect nature to have developed some safeguards? Wouldn't it be in out best interest to practice prevention in harmony with what nature already does? Can we use our natural intelligence to improve on our natural defenses? The answer to each of these questions is "yes."

USING THIS BOOK

This book is about prostate cancer prevention. Just as you wouldn't purchase an item in the store without first knowing a little about it, don't take each preventive step without first understanding why it's important and what it will do for you. Each chapter will give you that understanding, and explain how to put that knowledge to work for you every day.

1

Determine If You Have a Family History of Prostate Cancer

About 5 percent of cancers are directly caused by inherited genetic mutations; that means your chances of having inherited genes that will cause early prostate cancer are quite low. If you know you have such genes, early detection will be very important. Researchers agree that in the general population, other genes subtly increase cancer risk in concert with environmental factors. That means a man can have a tendency for prostate cancer, and other factors—which may or may not be within his control—can determine if and when the cancer will start.

Environmental factors include a multitude of controllable conditions, from the air we breathe and the food we eat, to the grade of gasoline we pump into our fuel tanks and spill on our hands, to the fumes we inhale when we sit in traffic or on a crowded airplane. Many factors affect how our genes are ultimately expressed over our lifetimes. For example, every study conducted on human fitness indicates that overweight men have a significantly greater prostate cancer risk. So, if you complete the genetic analysis recommended in this chapter and conclude that you have an above-average genetic risk, common sense indicates that you should exercise and keep your weight within the prescribed range.

THE FAMILY CANCER HISTORY

The only way to determine your general genetic risk is by doing a family cancer history. It is not difficult, can take as little as an afternoon, and can be very interesting. All you have to do is construct a family tree going back a generation or two. Try to write the age of each relative, whether male or female, if the relative had cancer, and if so, what type of cancer it was. Follow the example in Table 1.1 with Ron, a friend who has prostate cancer in his family.

From reviewing this chart of Ron's family, it appears that in recent generations about 40 percent of the family members experienced gender-related cancer. In a society where approximately 12.5 percent of men will get prostate cancer, Ron's family members have a greater risk. On both his mother's and father's sides, prostate cancer has occurred in men below the age of sixty. While sixty isn't a magic cutoff, it is a good marker for our purposes. Prostate cancer below age sixty is definitely not average; it suggests there is a minor genetic susceptibility lurking in Ron's family. Therefore, members of his family should take care to have regular exams and practice prevention.

In your own chart, look for several patterns that suggest a cause for concern, such as:

- Consistency. Is there a repeating pattern? A repeating pattern would be that one or two men in each generation developed prostate cancer going through all parents, grandparents, uncles, aunts, and cousins. Ideally, you could trace back to great-grandparents, great-uncles, and possibly even their siblings. Search for a consistent pattern of one or several men or women in each family with a gender-related cancer.

Table 1.1

Ron's Family Cancer Tree

Gender-Related Cancer

Ron and Siblings	Cancer Age	Parents and Siblings (Paternal P) (Maternal M)	Cancer Age	Cousins	Cancer Age	Grand-Parents and Siblings	Cancer Age	Great Grand-Parents and Siblings
Male 1		M-P		M-P	✓ 60	M-P	✓ 60	No health information
Male 2	✓ 45	M-P	✓ 55	M-P		M-P		
Male 3		M-P		M-P		F-P		
Female 1	✓ 52	M-P	✓ 48	M-P	✓ 44	M-M		
		M-M		F-P		M-M		
		F-M	✓ 53	F-P		F-M		
		F-M		M-M	✓ 53			
				M-M				
				F-M				
				F-M	✓ 62			

Cancer/Member

2/4	45	3/7	55	4/10	60	1/6	60	
	52		48		44			
			53		53			
					62			
50%		40%		40%		16%		

- Age. If a pattern seems to emerge, does an age pattern show up? Look at the gender-related cancers by decade; for instance, age forty to fifty, fifty-one to sixty, sixty-one to seventy. Does a consistent pattern emerge, such as between age fifty-one and sixty? If so, that is a significant finding. The older the age at which it occurs, the less serious the issue.

If a consistent pattern emerges in your family, review it by age. Although it is convenient to examine patterns decade by decade (for example, forty-one to fifty), you can categorize similarly by five-year increments. The younger a consistency displayed below seventy, the more concerned you should be.

Whatever results you find, however, don't panic! This is valuable knowledge and it puts you in control. You already know much more than the average person, and you have several courses of action. They all start with your doctor, and should include getting good responsible information.

WHAT TO TELL YOUR DOCTOR

Clean up your chart so it is clear and well organized, like Table 1.1, and show it to your doctor. Ask several simple questions, such as:

- Should I have a PSA test every six months? The PSA test for prostate cancer is most helpful when a pattern shows up (see chapter 2). In other words, let's say your test gives a reading of 0.8, which is very low and far below any risk. In another year, it goes to 1.2, which is within measuring accuracy, so it is still the same. Then, a year later it is 1.6, which is still far below the risk level of about 4; however, a trend is emerging. If the next test is 2.5, a trend is definitely established. You should see a urologist.
- Is genetic counseling appropriate? As our understanding of the role genetics plays in cancer has increased, the paramed-

ical professional specialty of genetic counselor has emerged. These counselors usually have advanced degrees and will examine your family history and assess your risk. A session with one of them can give you a good understanding of just how serious your risk is of prostate cancer.

Every man living in the United States right now has a one-in-eight chance of developing prostate cancer in his lifetime. If you took eight hundred men and followed them until they died at about age seventy-eight, one hundred would probably have evidence of prostate cancer at death. So, if your risk is about 10 percent above average, similar to Ron's family (say, one in seven), then you'd only have to follow seven hundred men to death at age seventy-eight to find one hundred with evidence of prostate cancer at death.

The reason I didn't suggest following eight men instead of eight hundred is that none or all of the eight might get prostate cancer. Statistics only work with large numbers, which brings us back to your family cancer tree. Unless your family is extremely large, the sampling is never big enough for average statistics to apply. That is where a genetic counselor enters the picture. Several patterns should raise some flags, such as:

- Is there a cancer pattern?
- Is the pattern age consistent?
  Below age fifty; a *bright* red flag should go up!
  Between fifty and sixty; a red flag should go up!
  Between sixty and seventy; a yellow flag should go up.
  Above age seventy; a pale yellow flag should go up.

A genetic counselor can help you to accurately and objectively assess these patterns.

2

Test for Early Detection: The Prostate Specific Antigen (PSA) Test

Testing for prostate cancer makes sense. Any prostate cancer detected early is confined to the gland; in short, it hasn't spread. The rate of survival under those conditions is almost 100 percent. The reason survival is so high is that the cancer can be removed, destroyed with radiation or chemotherapy, or, in some cases, treated in other ways. (Surprisingly, some forms of prostate cancer grow so slowly that if you're old enough, your best strategy might be to do nothing. That's right; you will not live long enough for the cancer to be a serious issue.) No matter what the treatment choice, you are better off if the cancer is detected as early as possible.

A TEST FOR EARLY PROSTATE CANCER DETECTION

The *prostate specific antigen* (PSA) is a protein produced only by the prostate gland. A normal prostate gland continually releases a very small amount of this protein into the bloodstream, so it generally appears in the blood in very low levels. Sensitive, routine tests can detect small amounts of PSA in the blood. By annually monitoring a man's PSA blood level to see if it becomes elevated, a doctor knows when something's gone awry.

Normal PSA in the most widely used routine test goes from 0.0 (none) to 4.0 (some). So, if your PSA is within that range, you shouldn't be concerned; simply repeat the same test in one year. Another less widely used test has an upper limit of 2.5. In both tests, the lab report will show a normal range for the type of test used. If the PSA is above the normal range, say, 5.0 or higher, you and your doctor should be concerned.

The test can actually show results into the hundreds, but most cancer is detected once the level exceeds about 10 but is less than 20. When a result above that range is received, the first thing you and your doctor should request is a second test. If a second test indicates the first report was accurate, you now have to know why it is elevated.

When the prostate is damaged, irritated, infected, or is cancerous, blood PSA levels are likely to be elevated. An elevated PSA level should raise your eyebrows because it indicates that all is not right, but it does not necessarily mean you have cancer. As other possibilities are ruled out, however, the risk that it is prostate cancer increases.

Several things can cause an elevated PSA, such as:

- Infection. A urinary tract infection can cause the prostate to become inflamed. Inflammation can cause an elevated PSA.
- Inflammation. A number of things can cause the prostate to be inflamed. Suppose you recently had some other urinary tract procedure, say, for kidney stones. This could easily irritate the prostate, cause inflammation, and elevate PSA.
- Rectal examination. For a long time the only prostate test was performed by the physician inserting his finger into the rectum and feeling the prostate. This procedure itself can

stimulate release of more PSA into the blood and cause an elevated test. It follows then that a sigmoidoscopy (test for rectal cancer, polyps, hemorrhoids, or other bowel problems) can similarly cause an elevated PSA.

- Enlarged prostate. The prostate continues growing throughout life, and some men simply have a larger prostate than others. More prostate tissue indicates more PSA, hence, a higher PSA blood test result.

Doctors can rule out infection or the results of a rectal exam, but once an elevated PSA persists, you should be referred to a urologist, who will make some further determinations.

Once you and your doctor suspect prostate cancer, there are several well-established courses of action. I recommend reading *Prostate Cancer: A Family Guide to Diagnosis, Treatment, and Survival* by Sheldon Marks, M.D. (available through Fisher Books, 555 West Massingale Road, Tucson, Arizona 85743-8416) to guide you through all the actions and procedures that will follow.

3

Eat to Reduce Risk

Most prostate cancer risk factors are related to diet, food, and nutrition. Food is the most controllable part of your entire environment. No one can make you eat foods that increase risk, and you can't be forced to eat foods that decrease your risk. Your dietary food and nutrition habits are 100 percent under your control.

Develop food selection habits that will promote and maintain good health while reducing your risk of heart disease, cancer, and the other degenerative diseases of aging. Some people are leery of nutrition advice because they envision losing the pleasure we all enjoy from food. Nothing could be more incorrect! The general food plan presented in this chapter provides all the variety and eating pleasure anyone could want, but also carries the bonus of better health. It is a modification of a general dietary plan commonly known as the Mediterranean Diet.

Governments, in the interest of maintaining a healthy population, generally develop food selection guides for their citizens to follow. These food policies are usually established by committees composed of dietitians; nutritionists; lobbyists representing industries such as dairy, meat, and selected agricultural farmers; medical groups; and myriad special interest groups that don't want their particular concerns ignored. The general guideline produced, if followed, will maintain a healthy citizenry. In the United States, it is administered by the Department of Agriculture.

There is another way to approach the same dietary objective. Look at populations that generally have above-average health and longevity and see what they tend to eat. It can be instructive to group common geographical locations together and allow any large ethnic and dietary differences to emerge. The World Health Organization (WHO) keeps mortality figures on prostate cancer in many countries; Table 3.1 shows these mortality rates together with comments on the prevalent diets in these areas.

Reviewing Table 3.1 and the comments in the right column make two things obvious:

Table 3.1

Prostate Cancer Mortality by Geographical Location

Location	Mortality Rate (Deaths/100,000)	Dietary Comments
Europe and U.K.	18.7	High meat, animal fat
U.S.A. and Canada	16.1	Mixed toward meat
Scandinavia	20.5	Animal fat, meat, dairy
Australia	19.0	Meat
Central America	16.5	Mixed, meat, animal fat
South America	17.0	Meat, animal fat
Baltic Republics and Poland	12.6	Processed meat
Mediterranean countries, including Israel	8.2	Mediterranean diet, tomato
Persian countries	5.5	More vegetarian, low-fat meat, vegetarian
Japan	5.1	Low meat, high fish and vegetarian, high soy
Korea	5.0	Lowest meat, high cruciferous, high soy

Source: Mortality data from WHO Mortality Database, 1999.

1. The more vegetarian the diet, the lower the prostate cancer mortality rate.
2. The more soy in the diet and the less meat, the lower the prostate cancer mortality rate. (More on the benefits of soy in the next chapter.)

Dietary trends among Mediterranean and Asian populations tend to fit these parameters, and these populations exhibit particularly good health patterns. This type of diet has become known as the Mediterranean Diet, but it could just as well be called the Optimum Health Diet. For our purposes, we'll refer to it as the Risk-Reduction Diet.

THE RISK-REDUCTION DIET
Monthly

Red meat

One serving monthly. A serving is about 3.5 to 4 ounces. That means that about once a month you could have meat as an entree; for example, a small steak, some roast beef, or a sensible-size hamburger. Alternatively, you might use a little meat as a condiment in a sauce with rice, or as a means of flavoring or adding texture to a dish. Meat as a condiment makes the most sense.

Weekly

The weekly part of the pyramid is far more varied than the monthly restriction and quite liberal.

Sweets

You may have desserts, such as cakes, candies, and cream pies, that have no redeeming nutritional aspects, about three to five times weekly, but not on a daily basis. In other words, sweets are somewhat special.

Eggs

This refers to eating visible eggs and doesn't consider eggs used in cooking and baking. The recommendation is three to five eggs weekly. As we'll see later, the best breakfast is cereal. This means that a man could have two eggs for breakfast about twice a week. Alternatively, a person could have cereal and one egg for breakfast several times a week.

Poultry

Broadly interpret this category to include waterfowl and you could have chicken, turkey, or duck about five times weekly. Rabbit and game, such as venison, can be included in this category if they aren't "corn fattened."

Daily

Fermented dairy products

This includes just about all dairy products except milk and ice cream (ice cream counts as about one-half serving). Cheese and yogurt should be used liberally. Also included in this group are some ethnic desserts, such as cannolis, which use ricotta cheese. Follow this diet plan studiously and you will have a little cheese daily as a snack, an appetizer, or even on crackers or bread as a light lunch; do the same with yogurt. Some societies say, "Always finish with cheese," and about 2 ounces of cheese are customarily served.

Olive oil

No, you don't sit down to a daily glass of olive oil. Rather, it is used liberally for salads, vegetables, sauces, some cooking, and always in place of butter. Put a little olive oil on a small dish and dip tasty bread in it, or drizzle it on the bread to accompany meals. Use canola oil in baking. Never use hydrogenated fat, lard, or butter.

Fruits

At least three servings should be eaten daily. A serving usually means an apple, pear, or orange; half a grapefruit; a cup of berries, such as blueberries, raspberries, or strawberries, or a slice of watermelon. Fruit should be a regular dessert; for example, a cup of sliced strawberries with sweetened yogurt is both a fermented dairy serving and a fruit serving. A 6-ounce glass of squeezed juice, such as orange, apple, or grape, is half a serving; an 8-ounce glass is a serving.

Beans and Legumes

Each day a single serving of legumes in some form should be eaten. Consider some examples: lima beans, string beans, cooked peas, black, red or kidney beans, chickpeas, garbanzos, or lentils. Whole bean soups, such as lentil soup or bean soup, or even refried beans (without fat) are good choices. Using soy milk on your morning cereal is half a bean serving. A "garden burger" or "harvest burger" is a bean serving; so is vegetarian sausage made from soy.

Vegetables

At least four vegetable servings daily, not counting those in soups and stews. A serving is two stalks of medium-sized broccoli with the florets, or a cup of sliced carrots, spinach, string beans, peas, or asparagus. The important thing to remember is it's better to have lots of servings and a wide variety.

Cereals, Grains, and Potatoes

At least six servings daily. Start each day with a cereal that delivers 5 or more grams of fiber per serving. A high-fiber cereal such as All Bran Bran Buds counts as two servings because it has about 13 grams of fiber. Half a cup of cooked corn, half a large potato or a whole medium one, a slice of whole-grain bread, or half a cup of wheat or other grain all count as a serving.

BUT DOES IT WORK?

Do people who eat this way have less cancer, heart disease, and diseases of aging?

Red Meat

Studies considering cancer risk as a function of meat consumption show some startling relationships. Meat consumption five times a week versus once monthly shows over a 3.5 times increased cancer risk; put another way, 350 percent. In contrast, we can compare people by ranking meat consumption in quarters. The highest versus the lowest 25 percent has 1.7 times the cancer rate; put more simply, 171 percent. These findings have held up in study after study; there is just no avoiding this conclusion.

The Mediterranean Diet

Diets have been compared on the basis of general diseases, such as heart disease and cancer and the degenerative diseases of aging. In general, every approach taken in research shows that a Mediterranean-type diet reduces risk by about 50 percent for most cancers (excluding female-specific cancers) and heart disease. More recent findings leave no doubt that it also reduces specific degenerative diseases, such as arthritis, cataracts, and bowel disorders. Interestingly, the research also indicates that it is never too late to start. In heart attack survivors who follow this general diet plan, heart attacks recur 30 percent less often compared to people who follow what is generally considered a good diet, but one that is far more liberal than the Mediterranean plan.

4

Soy

As discussed in chapter 3, getting more of your daily protein from vegetable sources, rather than from meat, reduces prostate cancer risk. For generations, most cultures have relied on soy and other vegetarian sources of protein, and much research has proven it's an excellent way to get adequate protein. Studies have shown repeatedly that soy foods have a special place in prostate cancer prevention.

SOY RESEARCH

Studying international rates of prostate cancer always brings scientists back to a few simple questions: Why do Asian men have 10 percent the prostate cancer rate of Western men? Why do some countries have even less than that? Why do Asian men who emigrate and adopt Western diets also adopt Western prostate cancer rates? One major reason, among others, is Asian men's dependence on soy-based foods for protein. Soy bioflavonoids, specifically isoflavones, are converted to other cancer-preventing substances by our intestinal flora.

Evidence for this reasoning comes from a number of different types of research, but no matter what method scientists follow, they end up with the same results. Cancer induced in laboratory animals is reduced in growth and proliferation by the addition of genistein and diadzein, the two isoflavones produced by soy. A few more advanced studies have even taken this approach to the genetic level; they go to the molecular basis of how the cancer gene is "turned on" and get the same results. Another technique has been to actually implant human prostate cancer cells in animals, then test whether genistein and diadzein inhibit tumor growth. (They do!)

Scientists aren't certain at this point how soy and other isoflavones work to prevent prostate cancer specifically. We can speculate, however, based on our knowledge of the mechanism by which they prevent other cancers. Testosterone, the male hormone, and its metabolites (materials produced as the hormone is broken down) cause the prostate gland to grow. They also increase the likelihood that a normal cell may become dysplastic and, finally, a cancer cell. For that conversion to happen, the metabolites must become attached to the cell. That is where soy and other isoflavones come into play. Part of the isoflavones resemble the structure of testosterone and testosterone metabolites. Hence, they can attach themselves to a prostate cell at the site where testosterone would attach and cause problems. If an isoflavone is there, the "bad stuff" cannot attach; consequently, risk is reduced.

While the mechanism for these results is not completely clear, there is no doubt about the effect; this is an area of very active research. To help prevent prostate cancer, you should change your diet to include more soy foods.

So, although the actual mechanism of action requires more research, the preventive effects are overwhelming. This is a compelling explanation for the low prostate cancer rates in populations with a high-soy protein diet.

PUTTING THIS KNOWLEDGE TO WORK

The admonition to simply "eat more soy" is too vague to be practical. The best studies prove quite clearly that 36 ounces of a soy beverage, such as soy milk, daily provides soy isoflavonoids comparable to levels that reduced prostate cancer induced in animals. What this tells us is that about one serving of soy daily, however, is probably sufficient when it is part of a prevention-oriented diet. The Mediterranean Diet emphasizes lots of vegetables, including beans and legumes, and fruits. Add to that at least one daily serving of soy food. This can include a variety of choices that range from soy burgers, 8 ounces of a soy beverage, tofu, and other soy foods. This is definitely a case of "more is better," so two or three servings are preferable to one.

Finding Soy Products

Soy protein products are available in most supermarkets and by catalog. One excellent catalog source is Harvest Direct, P.O. Box 4514, Decatur, IL 62525-4514; phone 1-800-835-2867.

Textured vegetable protein is the correct name for these products, which are usually made from purified soy protein. The protein is excellent in quality, low in fat, and contains none of the detrimental fats you'll learn about in chapter 12. It comes in several forms, as follows:

- "Burger/meat loaf" mix, when blended with water, is the equivalent of ground beef, which can be used to make hamburgers or a meat loaf. It comes in a variety of flavors— plain, Italian, or with herbs and spices. A seasoning mix can be purchased that even imparts the flavor of real breakfast sausage. I've served it often, and no one knew the difference.
- "Chicken" chunks are mixed with a small amount of water (a tablespoon of vinegar helps) to make chunks of excellent, imitation, white-meat chicken. This can be cooked and used in any recipe that calls for chicken. Note: Soy chicken chunks do require a little experimentation to get everything just right.
- "Beef" strips are hydrated in water and can be used whenever a recipe requires beef. In general, they can be cooked in stew, stroganoff, and chili, or after cooling, used in salad or as slices on a sandwich.

Soy products, such as Green Giant Harvest Burgers (they come in different flavors), The Original Garden Burger by Wholesome and Hearty Foods, Inc., and Morningstar Farms Breakfast Links by Worthington Foods, can be found in the frozen food section of the supermarket, and Westbrae Natural 1% Fat Lite Non Dairy Soy Beverage can be found on a shelf in the supermarket aisles. The soy beverage should be used whenever something calls for milk; for instance, on cereal, in shakes, and recipes.

SOY AND FIBER

Research has proven that dietary fiber is essential for the intestinal microflora to metabolize the soy isoflavones and bioflavonoids from most other foods into the materials the body readily uses. Therefore, it is very important to consume lots of dietary fiber so this process takes place. (We'll thoroughly explore dietary fiber in chapter 7.) Start tomorrow with a bowl of high-fiber cereal and try a soy beverage as a change from cow's milk. Put some fruit, especially fruit high in antioxidants, such as blueberries, sliced bananas, peaches, strawberries, or other berries, on your cereal. And remember that frozen fruit, thawed in the refrigerator, is just as nutritious as fresh fruit. Be sure to have some whole-pulp orange juice or grape juice, because these bioflavonoids help boost the antioxidant levels as well.

For snacks, eat a carrot or have an apple or an orange. All are excellent fiber sources, and they also provide good risk-reducing isoflavones and lignans.

At other meals, be sure to have at least one serving of beans, corn, or wheat, and don't forget a salad with lots of brightly colored peppers and green leaf lettuce.

5

Cruciferous Vegetables

Cabbage is the world's oldest cultivated vegetable. Different varieties of cabbage grow wild in all parts of the world and have been cultivated by every agricultural society. Cabbage and other cruciferous vegetables, especially mustard, have always been viewed as healthful foods and have formed the basis of many home remedies. At the dawning of the Christian era, some Roman communities banned physicians from practicing and declared people could stay healthy by eating cabbage. (Although medicine was primitive two thousand years ago, I'm not sure I would have dropped it entirely in favor of cabbage!) My mother fed me cabbage whenever I was sick.

The term *cruciferous* comes from the Latin for "to crucify" or "to place on a cross." The reproductive apparatus of cruciferous plants' flowers contains two components that nature has arranged like a cross. This consistent characteristic distinguishes them from all other plants.

All cruciferous vegetables provide a number of sulfur-containing antioxidants, the thiocyanates. As these foods are cooked or simply allowed to stand, these sulfur compounds change. As they change, they release materials that will tarnish silver, smell "musty," and taste pungent; this is why some people don't like these vegetables.

Mustard oil is produced by all these cruciferous plants and is used in various forms for medicinal purposes. One, the mustard plaster, is made of powdered mustard seed. When the powder is mixed with water, the chemical reaction produces heat and releases aromatic materials that help relieve nasal congestion. The objective of the plaster is to localize heat in the chest; a mustard plaster can generate enough heat to blister the skin unless a substantial layer of cloth is placed between the plaster and the skin. This heat helps stimulate circulation and loosen congestion, while the inhaled vapors from the oil attack the congestion from the inside. For years, the mustard plaster was one of the most effective remedies available for easing, if not curing, bronchitis and pleurisy.

People who eat cruciferous vegetables regularly have a much lower risk of many cancers, including cancers of the esophagus, stomach, colon, pancreas, lung, breast, skin, and prostate gland. Having an extra serving of coleslaw, snacking on radishes, or eating bok choy or brussels sprouts is good common sense.

Look at the list of sixteen common cruciferous vegetables below and you'll see that there are plenty from which to choose.

Broccoflower	Japanese horseradish
Broccoli	Kale
Brussels sprouts	Kohlrabi
Cabbage	Mustard
Cauliflower	Radish
Chinese cabbage (bok choy)	Rutabaga
Cress	Turnip
Horseradish	Watercress

There are over three thousand cruciferous plants, with many varieties in each group. For instance, there are over five common varieties of cabbage and over twenty varieties of radishes readily available in the United States alone. Cruciferous vegetables are raised in every part of the world where the climate permits green plants to grow. Each agricultural area has its own unique varieties.

CRUCIFEROUS VEGETABLES AND ANTIOXIDANTS

Green tea and cabbage have both been found to be protective against cancer. They are botanically unrelated, but they have two chemical constituents in common: phenols and indoles.

This poses a dilemma for scientists who are trying to determine the relative protective value of these natural materials. While these materials are present in all cruciferous vegetables, the exact amounts vary widely, and the amount in each vegetable is generally unknown. Like any natural foods, their composition differs by variety, location grown, climate, rainfall, and soil conditions.

Animal testing has proven that indoles, phenols, flavones, thiocyanates, and a few other components found in all cruciferous vegetables are protective against cancer. These naturally occurring chemicals in cruciferous vegetables and green tea are all antioxidants. If a chemist feeds an animal a combination of materials that produces both antioxidants and free radicals, the results show that these antioxidants prevent cancer.

Cruciferous vegetables are so consistently protective against cancer, however, that biochemists studied them in more detail. These studies indicate a property in these vegetables even more important to cancer prevention than their antioxidant qualities—their relationship with enzymes.

CRUCIFEROUS VEGETABLES AND ENZYMES

Enzymes are proteins that our bodies make to carry out chemical processes. Enzymes cause the same energy-yielding process to take place in your body as takes place in your car engine, but enzymes do it at body temperature rather than several hundred degrees. Your body extracts more energy, ounce for ounce, than your engine does, and produces exactly the same waste materials, carbon dioxide, and water. The enzymes act as catalysts, which make the process occur rapidly at body temperatures, but they themselves aren't changed in the process. In fact, enzymes are ready to process another batch of fat when the first one is done.

Biochemists who examined how body cells reacted to cruciferous vegetables found that cells produced new protective enzymes. I call them protective because they bring about destruction of materials that irritate cells and cause them to become dysplastic and then cancerous. Cruciferous vegetables cause each living cell to upgrade its own protective enzyme systems.

This process in which the number of enzymes increases as a result of an outside influence is known as *enzyme induction*. It means that the body cells make more of a particular enzyme in response to materials called *inducers*. In this case, inducers come from cruciferous vegetables. There may have been none or just a trace of a particular enzyme before the cruciferous vegetables came into play. After you eat the vegetables and absorb their material, your body cells start to produce a lot of that enzyme.

Induced protective enzymes fall into two classes: transferases and oxygenases. (The "ase" on the end of a word signals that it's an enzyme, if you're talking about a living system such as the human body.) Transferases transfer a toxic material to something else, such as beta-carotene, vitamin E, an indole, or some other antioxidant you took in from a vegetable or fruit. An oxygenase simply causes toxic forms of oxygen to be broken down in a way that's not destructive. In both cases, the toxin is neutralized.

Superoxide dismutase is one of the enzymes that our bodies produce in response to eating cruciferous vegetables. As its name implies, superoxide dismutase breaks down the toxic superoxide into pieces that are neutralized by other antioxidants, such as the carotenoids, vitamin E, indoles, and other antioxidants from vegetables, including the cruciferous vegetables.

Some of the toxic materials that are neutralized are those that attack genetic material in the nucleus of all body cells; this important fact provides the biochemical basis for the scientific observation that cruciferous vegetables seem to reduce the risk of all types of cancer. This is exactly what you'd expect from foods that have such broad effects—signaling every cell in the body. Protection by cruciferous vegetables seems to be almost universal.

I like to think of antioxidants and enzyme induction as the ultimate form of protection. Once the materials of protection are available, the body makes its own enzymes and uses them effectively. These enzymes go even further and use materials from the cruciferous vegetables to neutralize toxins. Our bodies then discard the neutralized toxins and are ready to take on more. To take advantage of this marvelous process, only one thing is asked of us: that we eat cruciferous vegetables regularly! How much simpler could our task be?

6

Garlic

Garlic is a perennial herb and a member of the lily family, which includes onions, chives, and leeks among its edible members. Garlic grows wild in Central Asia and has been cultivated for over five thousand years, making it one of the world's oldest cultivated plants.

Codex Ebers, a 3,550-year-old Egyptian medical papyrus, provided hundreds of therapeutic formulas, of which twenty-two used garlic. In 450 B.C., about one thousand years after *Codex Ebers,* Hippocrates considered garlic as one of the most important of his four hundred "simples," or therapeutic remedies. Among the therapeutic properties attributed to garlic in both *Codex Ebers* and Hippocrates' writings is its ability to stop tumors. Its use against tumors persisted throughout Asian and Western civilizations. In 1983, a paper appeared in an English medical journal entitled "Onion and Garlic Oils Inhibit Tumor Promotion." This first position paper, about 3,500 years after *Codex Ebers,* was the initial step in verifying whether garlic actually had tumor-inhibiting properties. Two lines of research have since verified that garlic does indeed have cancer-prevention and possibly even cancer-inhibiting properties.

One avenue of research pursued by many groups, most notably by a group led by Dr. Michael Wargovich in Houston, Texas, has studied garlic's ability to prevent and inhibit tumor growth in animals.

This research has indeed proven that garlic extracts do prevent cancer in animals given agents that normally induce cancer. Another approach, implanting human tumors in animals, has seen garlic extracts test out about as well as some chemotherapeutic agents used in cancer therapy.

Epidemiological studies support garlic's preventive qualities as well. Some studies, especially those examining digestive tract cancers (such as stomach cancer) have shown outstanding results. Garlic has also proven to have preventive effects on breast cancer. Prostate focus studies on garlic have not been conducted, but garlic definitely reduces general cancer risk in men. By coupling its gender-specific effects on breast and ovarian cancer with its general cancer risk reduction in men, one can surmise that it has a preventive effect on prostate cancer.

Garlic is a storehouse of antioxidants. Its active ingredient, allicin, imparts its odor and appears to be the source of its preventive qualities. You can prove for yourself how easily this material is transported throughout your body by doing a simple experiment: Have someone rub a peeled and crushed clove of garlic on the soles of your bare feet; in a few minutes you will taste garlic.

Most of what has been said about garlic also goes for onions, leeks, and other members of its botanical family, including asparagus. They all contain some allicin and its analogues—to a lesser extent than garlic, so they aren't as effective, but they contribute to the entire picture. Add chives to the sour cream on your potatoes, put a slice of onion on your salad, and add a crushed garlic clove to your pot of soup.

Experts tell me that Kyolic garlic sold as tablets in health food stores works as well as garlic. I'm skeptical, however, about artificially deodorized garlic tablets. Some active components have the pungent garlic odor, so it seems that if the odor is extracted by solvents, the effectiveness may be lost. I personally prefer to use fresh garlic, onions, leeks, chives, and asparagus.

GARLIC DO'S AND DON'TS

Do:

Add a clove of garlic to each serving of soup.
Add a clove of garlic to a garden salad.
Add a clove of garlic for each serving of fish, roast, or fowl.
Add a half clove of garlic for each serving of spaghetti sauce.

Don't:

Use garlic salt; it's salt.
Use deodorized garlic.
Use garlic oil, except when called for in a recipe.
Let a day pass without eating at least some garlic.

GARLIC'S OTHER HEALTH BENEFITS

Antibacterial

Garlic's antibacterial properties were first identified by the Egyptians. Nowhere were these properties more effective than during the great bubonic plague of Marseilles, France, in 1721. Smart criminals, forced to bury dead bodies, avoided the plague by making a concoction of garlic and vinegar or wine, which was quite effective against the plague-causing organisms. Garlic's antibacterial properties were used in World War I; wound dressings were often soaked in garlic oil, preventing infection and stopping it as well.

In 1944, Joseph Cavillito published a paper, which was followed by others through the early 1950s, verifying that garlic is about as good as penicillin against some microbes, and even against the common forms of yeast.

Heart Disease and Stroke

Garlic, eaten regularly and even when taken as tablets, reduces cholesterol. It must be used along with a low-fat, high-fiber diet to have the maximum effect, which isn't that spectacular. This practice has other benefits, however, which are not as easily measured.

Garlic's antioxidants reduce platelet aggregation. This factor causes several indirect effects that are quite important even if not widely known. The main effect is to reduce the risk of stroke and heart attack. Both these events involve the formation of an internal blood clot which is initiated when, for several reasons, the platelets *aggregate,* or form into a clump. Garlic reduces that probability.

Garlic also reduces blood viscosity. The result is that it helps to balance blood pressure, one of the major risk factors in heart disease and stroke.

7

Fiber

Prostate cancer is but one of the many modern health problems due in part to the continuing decline in the amount of dietary fiber we get in our diets. This fiber shortfall has come about with the proliferation of processed foods, our preference for fast food, and convenience eating. The results of inadequate fiber accumulate slowly, and a lifelong shortfall is insidious because its effects usually emerge when it's too late for correct dietary measures to have anything but a marginal influence. Indeed, fiber confirms more than any other nutrient that prevention is the best medicine—and nutrition is preventive medicine.

Increasing dietary fiber decreases prostate cancer risk; conversely, low dietary fiber increases prostate cancer risk.

WHAT IS DIETARY FIBER?

Dietary fiber is the undigestible part of plant foods; it passes through the stomach and small intestine without being digested. Each plant food has some dietary fiber. In addition to the major categories of cereals, grains, fruits, and vegetables, there are varieties within each group, such as red and bulgur wheat, Delicious and

McIntosh apples, and kidney and pinto beans, as well as many lesser-known foods. Each plant food has its own unique fiber content, so it is important to eat many different plant foods to obtain a wide variety of dietary fiber.

There are six general types of dietary fiber with hard, insoluble bran at one extreme, and gums at the other. There are many gradations between the two fiber extremes; most plants contain some of all of them, even though one type of fiber might predominate. Table 7.1 shows the availability and functions of each. We require fiber just as we need vitamins, but the body functions that call for fiber are far more subtle, so our dependence on fiber isn't as obvious.

Table 7.1

The Six Types of Fiber

Fiber Type	Water-Soluble	Function in Plant	Food Sources
Cellulose	No	Forms structure of cell walls with lignins	Wheat bran, fruit peels, seed coats
Lignin	No	Forms structure of cell walls with cellulose	Cereal grains, potato skins
Hemicellulose	Partly	Holds cells together with cellulose	Wheat bran, grains
Pectin	Yes	Binds cells together and holds water in fruit	Fruits
Gum	Yes	Binds stems, seeds, and vegetables	Oatmeal, vegetables, legumes
Mucilages	Yes	Binds seeds; binds stems in aquatic plants	Seaweed, seeds

While a vitamin deficiency seldom produces symptoms in less than one to three months, however, you'll probably know if you're not getting enough hard fiber within a day or so. Dietary fiber shortage also increases risk of diverticulosis, hemorrhoids, and varicose veins.

When you get enough correctly balanced fiber, it works for you in two ways: It corrects and prevents both watery and hard stools, and it produces firm but soft, easily moved stools. When you're getting the right amount and right mix of fiber, you'll move light brown stools once in twenty-four hours. That's why we call fiber "nature's regulator."

How much fiber produces correct regularity? Extensive research shows that the average 150-pound adult requires about 30 grams of fiber daily; you need about 25 grams if you weigh between 100 and 125 pounds, and 40 grams if you are around 200 pounds. About one-half to two-thirds of the fiber should be hard or insoluble fiber from grains and cereals, and the other third should be soft or soluble fiber from all plant foods. Emphasis should be placed on variety!

HOW FIBER WORKS

Think of a brush with specialized bristles that, in addition to moving things along, can selectively bind unwanted materials and remove them from the system. Each of the six types of fiber has properties we require. A varied diet provides them all. Of course, selective supplementation sometimes helps.

Hard fiber, the type found in wheat bran, is the "water carrier" that helps to produce good bowel movements. It gives good stool consistency and causes regularity. This fiber is found in all plant foods, but most abundantly in the high-fiber cereals, grains, most vegetables, beans, and tubers such as potatoes. You can't eat too much of these foods, and the results will be obvious as you increase them in your diet.

Soluble fiber, such as pectin, gums, saponins, and others, are the best at selective absorption. For example, pectin helps to reduce cholesterol by binding the bile acids produced by your liver from cholesterol and removing them in the stools. Oat bran does it even better, and guar gum better yet. Soluble fiber also binds the cholesterol and fat that we get in our diets and helps to carry them through the system.

Much research evidence proves that the soluble dietary fiber from fruits and vegetables can help remove unhelpful by-products of metabolism. This is because some materials produced by the body during this process are secreted into the intestine by the gallbladder for elimination and, in the absence of sufficient fiber, are reabsorbed.

Fiber and Detoxification

Over fifteen years ago, Dr. Ben Ershoff at the University of Southern California did some simple but very revealing experiments that have stood the test of time. He put laboratory rats on a basic diet and added a toxic material until the rats were barely surviving; then he added various types of fiber to this toxic diet, reasoning that fiber should bind up and neutralize the toxins and eliminate them from the body. The results were consistent. Some soluble fiber would detoxify the diet and restore growth completely. Other hard fiber, such as wheat bran, would partially restore growth, and some fiber, such as purified cellulose, had no detoxifying effect at all. Dr. Ershoff proved not only that fiber would make a toxic diet safe but also that some fiber bound unwanted materials—including carcinogens— better than others and that soluble fiber was most detoxifying.

Prostate cancer risk is elevated by toxic materials, which range from oxidizing agents derived from exhaust fumes to the by-products of testosterone metabolism. The body can remove these wastes (toxins) in two major ways: through urinary excretion and via stools. The first can be facilitated by maintaining a good fluid balance; the second, by maintaining adequate fiber intake.

Fiber is important because most metabolic wastes are either produced or processed via the liver. Some of these wastes are then
moved into the gallbladder and passed via the bile duct into the
large intestine. In the absence of adequate dietary fiber, a portion of
them are reabsorbed into the blood, increasing the body's cells' exposure to toxic effects. Adequate fiber and regular stools help to ensure their excretion. It's that simple!

Fiber and Water

Isoflavonoids are converted to prostate cancer–preventing by-
products by the intestinal microflora. Hard fiber, especially wheat
bran, is necessary for this transformation to take place.

Bran binds about nine times its weight in water. This material can
cause constipation if you don't get enough water; fiber in the absence of water can make stools dry, hard, and difficult to move. If
you ingest sufficient water and fiber in tandem, however, your stools
will be soft, consistent, and easily moved.

Our requirements for water and fiber extend far beyond simple,
good stool production, however. Water contains dissolved oxygen.
Many studies have shown that the most beneficial intestinal microflora are the *aerobes*; that is, microbes that thrive in the presence
of oxygen. When they thrive, the maximum by-products are produced. While bran is essential for correct regularity, its natural ability to bind water makes it a key, if subtle, player in prostate cancer
prevention.

FIBER FROM FOOD

An easy and practical way to get a good start on the fiber you need
is to begin each day with high-fiber cereal. Many excellent cereals
are available: Fiber One, All-Bran, Bran Buds, bran flakes, corn
bran, oat bran, oatmeal, and barley, to name a few. You can add
unprocessed bran to pancakes or waffles. Eat fruit on cereal, in

pancakes, or alone; eat fruit, vegetables, grains, and tubers at each meal. As your fiber intake improves, you'll become more regular. High-fiber snacks, such as carrots and fruits, are excellent all day, and remember to drink lots of water. Table 7.2 contains some readily available cereals that provide sufficient dietary fiber.

Table 7.2

Fiber from Cereals

Fiber per Serving	Cereals	
grams	Cold	Hot
3–5	Quaker Corn Bran	Quaker Oats
	Ralston Bran Chex	Malt-O-Meal
	Kellogg's Raisin Bran	Hot Wheat Cereal
	Generic/store brand	Ralston Cream of Wheat
	raisin bran	Wheatena
	Kellogg's Cracklin' Oat Bran	Unprocessed bran
	Kellogg's Bran Flakes	Miller unprocessed bran
	General Mills Raisin	Quaker unprocessed bran
	Nut Bran	
	Post Fruit 'N Fiber	
	Post Bran Flakes	
	Post Natural Raisin Bran	
9	Kellogg's All-Bran	
	Nabisco 100% Bran	
Over 12	Kellogg's All-Bran	
	Extra Fiber	
	General Mills Fiber One	

SHOULD YOU TAKE FIBER SUPPLEMENTS?

I'm often asked, "How do I know I'm getting enough fiber?" My answer is, "You should have an easy bowel movement every twenty-four hours and always within thirty-six hours. The stools should be well formed, their color should be light brown, and preferably about 10 percent will float."

If you're eating according to the dietary plan in chapter 3 and your stools still don't fit that profile, start using a good fiber supplement. Fiber supplements are usually made from psyllium hulls (psyllium provides mucilage that helps to bulk the stools and maintain regularity) and are often sold as "natural vegetable laxatives" under store brand names. Mix up to 1 full tablespoon with water and drink it about thirty minutes before a meal.

Other fiber supplements, such as fiber wafers and high-fiber crackers and cookies, can be simply eaten as food.

A DAY WITH 35 GRAMS OF FIBER

Most people have difficulty understanding how 25 to 35 grams of fiber intake daily is achieved, so I've prepared Table 7.3. This "Day of Fiber" exceeds what most people require; it would be sufficient for a 200-pound man.

This guide allows for many substitutions. For instance, beans and rice make an excellent protein entrée that also provides fiber. That combination could easily substitute for a luncheon sandwich.

You cannot get too much dietary fiber. In the past thirty years, I've never observed or read about a study in the medical literature in which people have consumed too much dietary fiber—and that includes one study in which the volunteers took in 90 grams daily.

Table 7.3

A Day with 35 Grams of Fiber

Food Item	Soluble	Insoluble	Total	Calories
Breakfast				
Bran flakes	1.0	4.0	5.0	121
(with ½ cup skim milk)				93
½ grapefruit	0.6	1.1	1.7	39
Snack				
Banana	0.6	1.4	2.0	105
Lunch				
2 slices wheat bread	0.6	2.2	2.8	122
Corn (½ cup)	1.7	2.2	3.9	89
Broccoli	1.6	2.3	3.9	23
Peach (dessert)	0.6	1.0	1.6	37
Snack				
Apple	0.8	2.0	2.8	81
Dinner				
Brussels sprouts	1.6	2.3	3.9	30
Small salad	1.6	2.2	3.8	50
Potato	0.7	1.0	1.7	200
Melon (dessert)	0.4	0.6	1.0	130
Snack				
Pear (crispy)	0.5	2.0	2.5	98
Total	**12.3**	**24.3**	**36.6**	**1218**

Other foods eaten during the day	Calories
Yogurt, low-fat	228
Fish	150
Turkey slices	100
Spreads and condiments	100
Total calories	**578**
Total daily calories	**1796**

Note: This day is designed to provide enough fiber with flexibility. There's room to have other desserts or accompaniments, such as wine, up to 1,800 calories for women and 2,200 calories for men.

8

Always Have Color on Your Plate

"Always have color on your plate" is an old wives' saying that means one should include green, yellow, and red vegetables with every meal. Folk wisdom can be as good as modern science because it has survived the test of time. This particular bit of advice is more important in preventing prostate cancer than any other single statement. It ensures that people get enough carotenoids for their bodies to make vitamin A, with more left over to do what carotenoids do best—prevent cancer.

Carotenoids are pigments that impart color to plants and are important for plant growth and survival. At last count, there were 563 known carotenoids classified into ten groups, and chemists expect to find even more. Beta-carotene and other carotenoids are always associated with a specialized green pigment called chlorophyll. Both carotenoids and chlorophyll are found in a plant's leaves or other green tissues exposed to sunlight. Carotene pigments are also found in roots, stems, flowers, fruits, and even in animal tissues. For instance, flamingos, salmon, and lobsters eat plants that contain carotenoids. These pigments accumulate in flamingo feathers, salmon flesh, and lobster shells and give them their distinctive colors.

If you eat lots of carrots every day for a month or so, you might notice the palms of your hands turning a little orange; it's beta-carotene accumulating in your skin.

Free radicals and superoxides are highly reactive materials that only survive for milliseconds; that's 0.001 of a second. They come in many forms; some are created when sunlight strikes normal, everyday chemicals, such as oxygen. Others arise from chemical reactions involving such commonly occurring chemicals as chlorine in water, carbon monoxide or nitrogen oxides in exhaust fumes, and countless others. We call some of these toxins superoxides because they contain an especially lethal and reactive form of oxygen. Free radicals have an electric structure that makes them especially reactive, too. Although they only survive for a tiny fraction of a second, they react so readily with everything that they take oxygen's place in the chemical reaction oxidation. The result is oxidative destruction. Think of them as microscopic explosives that can destroy delicate biological structures, such as cell membranes or nuclei.

All carotenoids have an abundance of internal structures that react easily with these superoxides, free radicals, and the toxins they produce. The carotenoids neutralize them, and they can be safely excreted from the body. Not only do carotenoids act as nature's sunblock, they also prevent noxious materials from destroying sensitive tissues.

Plants use different carotenoids as they grow and mature. For example, two carotenoids abundant in tomatoes, lycopene and beta-carotene, filter different parts of light. Beta-carotene is the most effective carotenoid for protecting the tomato when it's green and still undergoing photosynthesis. Then, when photosynthesis is no longer occurring, lycopene takes over and protects the tomato against other toxins. The emergence of lycopene—the red color—also announces that the tomato is ripe.

Each carotenoid works most effectively at a specific temperature. Egg yolks rely on beta-carotene and canthaxanthin. Because the temperature changes inside an egg as it incubates, it's important to have protectors that function at the temperatures and conditions likely to be present. Beta-carotene protects better at lower temperatures than canthaxathin does. Both carotenoids come from chicken feed the egg-laying hen eats and give the yolk its color.

VITAMIN A

Vitamin A is essential for the development of all tissue but is especially critical for eye tissue. Vitamin-A deficiency in underdeveloped countries accounts for at least sixty thousand cases of permanent childhood blindness annually. When there is not enough beta-carotene or vitamin A in young children's diets, eye tissues become keratinized. Keratinized tissue looks like a callous on your hand or foot, not like clear, normal eye tissue. Obviously, you can't see out of a keratinized eye. This blindness can be prevented with a few cents' worth of beta-carotene or vitamin A, but once keratinized tissue becomes established, it can't be reversed. Preventing blindness for the whole world annually would be possible at only a fraction of the cost of a single military aircraft.

What vitamin A does for your eye development, it does for all body tissues throughout your life. These functions are all part of its role as a vitamin; therefore, vitamin A is necessary for life. It's essential for all cell growth and development; it helps all body processes work by directing each cell to fill its intended role. For example, the cornea cells of your eye are clear and transparent, while a cell in your intestines is long and slender and produces mucus; yet, they begin as the same kind of basic, undifferentiated cell. Vitamin A triggers the change. For example, our intestinal cells reproduce so rapidly that they're completely replaced about every three weeks. Vitamin A is absolutely essential for this process to occur correctly; and this is similarly true for all the fifty trillion cells in our bodies.

Vitamin A is also required for a strong immune system that correctly identifies and kills foreign germs and cancer cells. In short, we can't live without vitamin A.

Some carotenoids are about 50 percent effective as sources for vitamin A, and others (for example, lycopene) aren't effective at all. Of the 563 carotenoids, beta-carotene is the most efficient source of vitamin A.

DAILY BETA-CAROTENE REQUIREMENTS

The average North American dietary intake is less than 6 milligrams of beta-carotene per day; 6 milligrams daily simply isn't enough. Many experts say we should strive for a minimum of 15 milligrams of beta-carotene daily. If you live and work in a city, use public transportation, are exposed to smoke and fumes, exercise heavily where you might be exposed to fumes, or expose your skin to the sun, you definitely need more carotenoids.

As Table 8.1 shows, you can get 15 milligrams of carotenoids daily with little effort. It's as easy as following these daily rules:

- Eat a serving of red or orange vegetables every day; two servings is better and cooked is better than raw.
- Eat two green leafy vegetables every day.
- Eat a piece of fruit with colored flesh every day.
- When in doubt, supplement. Use 5 to 15 milligrams of beta-carotene, depending on your diet.

Table 8.1

Good Food Sources of Carotenoids

Vegetables	Milligrams of Carotenoids per ½ cup serving	Fruits	Milligrams of Carotenoids per ½ cup serving
Avocado	0.9	Apricots	1.7
Beet greens	2.2	Cantaloupe	3.1
Broccoli	0.9	Cherries	0.6
Cabbage	1.3	Loquats	1.0
Carrots	12.0	Mandarin orange	0.6
Chard, Swiss	1.6	Prunes	1.0
Chicory	2.2	(10 prunes)	
Collards	3.0	Mango	4.8
Dandelion greens	3.6	Nectarine	0.6
Dock	2.1	Papaya	3.7
Kale	2.3	Peaches	0.5
Lamb's-quarters	5.2	Persimmon	2.2
Mustard greens	1.3		
Mustard spinach	4.4		
Spinach	5.0		
Spring onions	1.5		
Peppers (sweet red)	2.0		
Pokeberry	4.3		
Pumpkin	16.0		
Seaweed (Nori)	3.1		
Squash (winter)	2.2		
Squash (hubbard)	3.7		
Swamp cabbage	1.9		
Sweet potato	16.8		
Red tomato	1.0		
Tomato paste	2.0		
Turnip greens	3.1		

9

Tomatoes

Tomatoes are the most widely eaten vegetable in North America (although technically, they are fruits). Early Spanish explorers discovered them among the native food plants of South America. Once the explorers brought back the tomato seeds, tomatoes were cultivated in Europe and England as ornamental plants. The fruit, a berry, was avoided by some as the "forbidden fruit" of Genesis. Its use, however, was accelerated by others who saw tomatoes as the aphrodisiac that had aroused Adam. Aphrodisiac users prevailed and tomatoes soon became known as "love apples." By the 1600s, they were being eaten in salads, although their use was not widespread for another two hundred years.

Tomatoes prove that vitamin and mineral content is not the only criterion for selecting food. Tomatoes rank sixteenth in vitamin and mineral content, but they are number one in actual use because of their flavor, mouth feel, appearance, and ease of eating. Broccoli is clearly number one in nutritional content, but it is actually number sixteen in popularity.

Men who eat tomatoes five times weekly, especially as tomato sauce or soup from puree, are 50 percent less likely to develop prostate cancer than men who don't. (This fact is yet one more reason to follow the modified Mediterranean Diet plan described in chapter 3.) A good approach is to use tomato sauce on pasta, beans, vegetables, fish, and other compatible foods.

Tomatoes showed up in many epidemiological studies as being preventive, first in bladder cancer, then in prostate cancer. By statistical analysis, the protective effect exhibited by tomatoes was narrowed down to lycopene, the red carotenoid pigment in tomatoes, watermelon, and other bright red fruits and vegetables.

There are no lycopene supplements available for those who don't like tomatoes. Lycopene levels in the body don't remain elevated for long periods. It is also difficult, if not impossible, to purify and provide sufficient lycopene in a simple pill or capsule. In addition, we're not sure it's actually the lycopene delivering these protective benefits. It could be a unique combination of lycopene and some obscure bioflavonoid. Common sense dictates that a tomato, watermelon, or strawberry has more than lycopene; it could be a combination of several or many carotenoids together at the same time that makes it effective.

The findings on tomatoes support the folk wisdom "always have color on your plate" discussed in chapter 8. Indeed, studies suggest that tomatoes, tomato sauces, and tomato soups, as well as watermelon and other red fruits and vegetables, are more important than we might have expected. A plate of spaghetti with tomato sauce served with watermelon for dessert is a protective powerhouse against several types of cancer, especially prostate cancer.

COOKED OR RAW?

Cooking vegetables probably reduces vitamin-C content and possibly one or two other vitamins, but it actually makes most antioxidants, especially the carotenes, more available to the body. Extensive testing by food scientists has proven that your body absorbs more lycopene from tomato sauce than from an equivalent amount of raw tomatoes. This has been similarly demonstrated for most nutrients. The reason for this seeming paradox is the fiber matrix.

Fiber doesn't come in vegetables in a form that is easily released. After all, it gives the plant its structure and in some cases, it protects essential materials. For example, the coat of an apple seed lets it pass through the body completely undigested. So, this fiber matrix can be tough enough to withstand the entire digestive system.

When vegetables are cooked, the matrix—we see it as fiber—breaks down slightly and the nutrients that are enrobed within the matrix are more easily released for good absorption.

Food scientists have compared nutrient and antioxidant availability from cooked and uncooked vegetables and there is simply no contest; cooked wins hands down every time. This doesn't mean you should cook all vegetables to mush. Just cook them lightly so they are still somewhat crunchy, but a little soft.

10

Establish Habits That Decrease Risk

Even though the practices outlined in this chapter aren't specific for a single cancer, they seem to always show up missing in people with high cancer risk. They are the habits I encourage my family and friends to establish themselves. People who follow these recommendations usually have a lower cancer risk than people who don't.

EAT BREAKFAST

"Breakfast is the most important meal of the day." This folk wisdom is absolutely correct. When people skip breakfast, they usually don't meet their daily fiber requirements, especially for hard wheat fiber. Fiber is so essential that I've devoted chapter 7 to it. Sure, you can take fiber supplements and get it from fruits and vegetables, but skip breakfast and you're not likely to get enough essential hard fiber.

Breakfast often begins with a glass of juice, fruit, or better still, both. So, by skipping breakfast, you'll probably also miss citrus fruit and some important antioxidants, especially the citrus bioflavonoids. Citrus isoflavonoids are antioxidant risk reducers by themselves, and some are converted to materials that seem to lessen gender-specific cancers, such as prostate cancer.

Sliced bananas, a cancer risk reducer, are often a topping for cereal. Bananas, like soy, provide isoflavonoids, which, when acted on by healthy intestinal microflora, reduce cancer risk.

Few men regularly drink soy beverages. Take chapter 4 seriously and begin using soy milk on your cereal. Skip breakfast, and you're less likely to get this nutritious beverage and the protection it imparts. Later in the day, a chocolate soy beverage can be very refreshing.

SKIP THE DONUT OR COFFEE CAKE

A coffee break in the morning and afternoon is such a well-established institution that unions often negotiate it into contracts. Some offices have a room where employees can get a freshly brewed cup of coffee, and in others, coffee is delivered so you don't have to leave the office. Unfortunately, snacks taken with coffee are usually empty-calorie foods, loaded with unhealthy omega-6 oils and fat, such as cakes and cookies.

While there is no evidence indicating that coffee increases any cancer risk, there is data showing that tea (made from tea leaves) is a risk reducer. Fruits and vegetables, excellent preventive snacks, don't taste good with coffee, but they do with tea. So the "coffee break" tradition is an insidious factor promoting high-fat, empty-calorie foods such as donuts and sweet rolls. Switching to tea can make fruit and vegetables more palatable and convert this "break" into a preventive opportunity. So drink tea, not coffee, to reduce risk.

SKIP FAST-FOOD LUNCHES

Just ten years ago, most burgers had a single patty. Now many people eat larger, double burgers, fries, and a soft drink for lunch because it's inexpensive, fast, and easy to eat on the run. Eating like this more than once monthly, however, increases the specific risks of colorectal cancer, non-Hodgkin's lymphoma, and prostate cancer. How many people eat like that every day? Twice a day? With just a little effort, you may be able to find places that sell veggie burgers; try them and make fast food healthy food.

In some dietary surveys, researchers found that about 30 percent of the vegetables people consumed were French-fried potatoes. It's important to eat at least three servings of vegetables daily, but French fries don't count. Potatoes are an excellent food and provide complex carbohydrates, a little fiber, and vitamins and minerals, especially when they're eaten with the skin left on, such as baked or boiled. French fries aren't inherently bad in moderation, but the oil used in frying adds an excessive amount of calories for the nutrition the potatoes deliver—and fries are likely to displace a salad, side of cole slaw, or a more nutritious vegetable such as broccoli.

DON'T MAKE RED MEAT THE CENTER OF YOUR MEAL

To many people, a meal isn't complete if it lacks beef. Historically, serving beef was a way of displaying wealth and hospitality. The quest for more tender and tasty beef led to fattening cattle in feedlots where they were fed corn and other grains to increase their weight and fat content. This change in the cattle-raising process made high-fat beef cheap, tasty, and easy to eat. It is not uncommon for many people to eat half a pound of beef at a meal or in a single day.

WASH YOUR PRODUCE

We're always told that pesticides are safe. If they are, why do chemists who work with them have higher cancer rates? Although the evidence is not all in, there's enough for all practical purposes to realize some common sense should prevail. Always wash fruits, vegetables, and other produce with a little dish detergent and rinse them well. This will eliminate the surface chemicals.

11

Increase Your
Antioxidant Intake:
Vitamins C and E
and Selenium

Scientists have confirmed that vitamins C and E along with the mineral selenium afford some prostate cancer prevention. This is not surprising to anyone who understands diet, biochemistry, and how antioxidants work.

Glutathione peroxidase destroys free radicals and superoxides. Its name means that it destroys peroxides (the potent oxidants that form in tissues) and uses glutathione as a helper. Glutathione requires selenium to function; and wherever selenium is at work, vitamin E can't be far away because they function together. Vitamin C enters the prevention picture because it acts as a glutathione recycler. When the glutathione peroxidase destroys a peroxide, the glutathione becomes deactivated. At this point, vitamin C regenerates the glutathione.

A second role for this nutrient team is its involvment in other metabolic processes such as maintaining good immune function and keeping potential inflammation in check.

When people learn that vitamins C and E and selenium show up as preventive nutrients, they often ask, "How much should I take?" While research indicates that getting these nutrients somewhat above the RDI (Recommended Daily Intake) is preventive, it doesn't yield precise levels. It suggests, however, that prevention is maximized at about 300 milligrams of vitamin C, about 100 international units (I.U.) of vitamin E, and about 50 micrograms of selenium.

VITAMIN C

You can get that 300 milligrams of vitamin C by simply eating extra fruit. For instance, eating oranges (three to four), strawberries (three to four), and kiwi fruit (four), or drinking extra orange juice (two and a half glasses) during the day will deliver approximately 300 milligrams of vitamin C. And it wouldn't hurt to take a 500 milligram vitamin-C supplement; unneeded vitamin C is simply excreted by the body.

VITAMIN E

Vitamin E is a different story. It is difficult to eat a diet that provides more than about 15 to 30 international units of vitamin E. So, sensible supplementation is necessary. Studies indicate that vitamin E is safe even at 3,000 I.U. No one needs to take that much, however.

Eight materials provide vitamin E activity: four tocopherols and four close cousins, the tocotrienols. The best source for these materials is wheat germ oil, but they're also found in soy, corn, peanuts, walnuts, and sunflower and other seeds, as well as most vegetables.

Seed oils are also found in the flesh of animals that eat these foods. We don't know for sure if vitamin E's protective effect is imparted by one of these materials or by several working together, so it makes sense to obtain all of them from natural food sources. Table 11.1 on pages 56 and 57 lists good dietary vitamin-E sources.

SELENIUM

Selenium is yet another story. It is clearly safe up to 300 micrograms daily, and there is no need to go above that level. (Like other nutrients, the daily requirements would not cover a dot on this page.) Selenium levels show a U-shaped correlation with prostate cancer. In other words, both low and high blood levels of selenium increase risk. This simply means that we need enough selenium to maintain good health, yet too much can be dangerous. A practical compromise is to use a supplement that provides 100 I.U. of vitamin E (up to 400 I.U. would be fine), and about 50 micrograms of selenium.

Table 11.1

Vitamin E Content of Foods

Food	Vitamin E, in milligrams
Fats and Oils	
(Serving size is 1 tablespoon)	
Wheat germ oil	20
Sunflower oil	6
Safflower oil	5
Cottonseed oil	5
Almond oil	5
Corn oil	3
Olive oil	2
Peanut oil	2
Canola oil	3
Other oils provide about 0.5 milligram per serving.	
Nuts and Seeds	
(Serving size is 1 ounce)	
Almonds, dried	7
Almonds, oil roasted	2
Brazil nuts, dried	2
Hazelnuts, dried	7
Peanuts, dried	3
Peanut butter	6
Pistachios	2
Other nuts provide about 0.5 milligram per ounce.	
Cereals	
(Serving size is 1 ounce)	
Oatmeal	1
Cornmeal	1
Wheat cereal (whole wheat)	1
Unprocessed cereals provide about 0.5 milligram per serving. Highly processed cereals provide considerably less.	
Baked Goods and Confections	
Apple pie, ⅛ pie	7
Blueberry pie, ⅛ pie	7
Pound cake, 3½ ounces	3
Chocolate bar	2
Chocolate cookie, 1	2

Food	Vitamin E, in milligrams
Spreads	
(Serving size is 1 tablespoon)	
Margarine	
Mazola, regular or unsalted	8
Mazola, diet	3
Mustard	1
Mayonnaise	
Hellmann's	11
Soybean	3
Peanut butter, Skippy	2
Other spreads provide about	
0.5 milligram per tablespoon.	
Grain Products	
(Serving size is 1 cup unless specified)	
Whole-wheat bread (2 slices)	1
Macaroni	1
Spaghetti	1
Wheat germ (toasted), ¼ cup or 1 ounce	6
Other grain products provide about	
0.5 milligram per serving.	
Fruits	
Mango, 1 medium	2
Apple, medium with skin	1
Other fruits provide less than 0.5 milligram per serving.	
Vegetables	
(Serving size is ½ cup unless specified)	
Asparagus, 4 spears	1
Avocado, 1 medium	2
Sweet potato, 1 medium	6
No other vegetables provide 1 gram of vitamin E.	
Fish, Meat, Poultry	
(Serving size is 3½ ounces)	
Chicken, turkey, most fowl	1
Salmon and oily fish	2
Shrimp, scallops, shellfish	3
Beef liver	1
Other meats and nonoily fish provide about	
0.5 milligram per serving.	

12

Cancer-Preventing Fats

The belief that "fish is brain food" has been held around the world for well over two thousand years. Fish supplies omega-3 oils, and among them is docosahexaenoic acid (DHA), essential for brain and eye tissue development (specifically the retina) in infants; it remains fundamental to those tissues throughout life. Current research focuses on these oils—often woefully short, if not deficient, in modern diets—as one cause of attention deficit disorder. Once more, modern research is validating folk wisdom—fish really is brain food. Now new findings are suggesting that the oils found in fish also help prevent cancer.

In 1980, a Scandinavian medical journal published an extensive decade-long study comparing the health and diet of Greenlanders to their counterparts in Denmark. Greenlanders and Danes share the same Nordic background and a similar genetic makeup, so they are a homogenous population. Over the centuries, diets of both groups have remained high in fat, but the fat composition was quite different because of its sources. Other dietary levels, such as protein and carbohydrate, weren't significantly different between the two groups.

Many diseases, especially inflammatory diseases, were almost or completely nonexistent among the Greenlanders. Breast cancer was conspicuously absent, and other cancers, including prostate cancer, were very low! Danes on the other hand, have the same cancer rates as people in most Western countries.

What was it that protected Greenlanders from breast and other cancers? Some factors, of course, are obvious; for instance, lack of pollution. A less obvious factor uncovered in the research was the type of dietary fat prevalent in their diets.

Table 12.1 describes some of the different types of fat. The Greenlander's main protein sources are cold-water fish and marine mammals (whales, sea lions, and so on), which are rich in the omega-3 oils and also contain some omega-6 oils. In contrast, Danes, like people in most Western countries and especially North America, get their protein from meat that provides almost exclusively omega-6 oils.

When the ratio of omega-6 to omega-3 oils in tissue and blood is measured, Danes have a ratio that is eleven times greater in blood fat and seventeen times greater in tissue fat. This means that compared to Greenlanders, Danes have very little omega-3 oils in their tissues.

Similar comparisons have been made among other peoples with similar results; for example, between Japanese and Americans, seacoast Japanese and Japanese city dwellers, Canadian Arctic dwellers and people living on the border of the United States and Canada, and people in Seattle, Washington, who eat fish versus people in the Midwest who don't. The outcome is always similar. Body tissues reflect diet; you really are what you eat!

Scientists have concluded that omega-6 oils are not involved in cancer initiation, but once it is established, they're involved in its growth or, more scientifically, its promotion. In contrast, the omega-3 oils seem to inhibit cancer cell growth, but they do not prevent the cancer's initiation.

Look at it this way: once cells have entered the dysplastic phase as discussed in previous chapters, the omega-6 oils seem to promote their transition into full-blown cancer cells, while the omega-3 oils seem to inhibit this transition.

Table 12.1

Types of Fat

Fat	Abbreviation	What It Is
Fat	None	A food substance that provides 9 calories per gram or 252 calories per ounce.
Hard Fat	None	A fat that is hard at room temperature, such as the "white" fat around beef, or butter. Crisco is a good commercial example.
Oil	None	A fat in liquid form at room temperature that provides 9 calories per gram (for example, corn oil).
Fatty Acid	FA	The smallest unit of all fats and oils. The term acid refers to its structure.
Saturated Fat or Saturated Fatty Acid	SFA	A fat consisting of fatty acids that have no open (unsaturated) regions. Usually solid at room temperature (solid animal fat; for example, beef).
Monounsaturated Fatty Acid	MFA	An oil with one open (unsaturated) area on its fatty acids. Heavy liquid at room temperature, such as olive oil.
Polyunsaturated Fat or Polyunsaturated Fatty Acid	PUFA	An oil with many open (unsaturated) areas on its fatty acids. Light in color and liquid at room temperature. The more unsaturated, the lighter the liquid (for example, safflower oil versus olive oil).
Omega-3 Oil or Omega-3 PUFA	O-3	A PUFA in which the unsaturated areas are in a unique location, the third bond from the omega end.
Omega-6 Oil or Omega-6 PUFA	O-6	A PUFA in which the unsaturated areas are in a unique location, the sixth bond from the omega end.
Essential Fatty Acids or Essential Oils	EFA	PUFAs that are essential for human health, if not life itself. We must get some O-3 and O-6 oils in our diets.

The biochemical foundation for this consistent observation can be inferred from research on inflammatory diseases, such as rheumatoid arthritis. Omega-6 oils are metabolized to substances that promote tissue oxidation. Similar metabolites from the omega-3 oils do not, however. This makes an enormous difference in tissue damage in an inflammatory disease, but is almost impossible to evaluate in cancer research. It is one more piece of compelling circumstantial evidence, though, that cannot be dismissed.

After cancer has started, the omega-3 oils seem to exert a controlling influence that slows tumor growth. Currently there is speculation that this is due to the conversion of a single omega-3 oil to hormonelike substances called prostaglandins, and other substances, the leukotrienes. Most researchers conclude that this is why omega-3 oils help prevent cancer, while omega-6 oils are, at best, neutral and, at worst, modestly promote it. It is all in the balance of the prostaglandins and leukotrienes from oils. The answer will probably require another decade of research.

FAT AND OIL USE AND CANCER

In Mediterranean countries, people use olive oil in place of butter, corn oil, and other cooking oils. They dip bread in olive oil instead of using butter or margarine. Olive oil and vinegar, with appropriate herbs, is their salad dressing. Olive oil is what we call a monounsaturated MFA oil. It contains some PUFA (and even some of that is omega-3), but its major component is a monounsaturated oil called oleic acid. Scientists have proven that MFAs are neutral with respect to heart disease, and that they reduce breast cancer risk.

In Western countries, butter and margarine are traditionally used as a spread and for cooking. Beginning in the 1960s, however, Westerners were weaned from saturated fat to the notion that the lighter the oil, the greater its PUFA content, and the better it was for you. So, corn, sunflower, and safflower oils, among other light oils, became the norm in both spreads and cooking. In summary, omega-6 oils became the most popular oil used.

Our shift from saturated fat to polyunsaturated fat was instigated by widespread concern about heart disease. The idea was that we could keep eating a high-fat diet if the fat in the diet was a little better for us. Because the only nutritional concern was cholesterol, this notion seemed like a good one—at the time. Now, we know better. Total fat from all sources should be cut back, and we need omega-3 oils in more abundance than anyone had previously thought.

In contrast to Western populations, Asian peoples use soy oil for just about everything: cooking, salad dressing, and even for spreads—and soy oil has a reasonable omega-3 oil content. Moreover, in Japan and other Asian countries, dietary fat provides only about 15 to 20 percent of calories, in contrast to 35 to 40 percent of calories in Western countries. Since total fat content has a role in cancer, this is one more reason why the cancer rate is much lower in Asian countries.

GETTING THE RIGHT FATS THROUGH DIET

Ten to 15 percent of your total daily calories undoubtedly come from protein. Typically, people think of meat when they think "protein." Start thinking of fish when you think protein and increase your intake of omega-3 oils by starting to eat more fish. A simple comparison will make the point.

Ground chuck provides 32 percent of its calories from protein, with 66 percent from fat. All the PUFA in beef is omega-6. Salmon derives 67 percent of its calories from protein and 28 percent from fat, with about 2 grams of omega-3 oils. If you could simply eat salmon daily, you would reduce your total fat intake and increase your omega-3—probably from almost none to a lot.

Table 12.2 lists commonly available fish with total PUFA content and the amount of omega-3 oil delivered in a typical $3\frac{1}{2}$-ounce serving. You don't need a degree in nutrition to recognize that you can increase your daily omega-3 oils by simply selecting fish for one meal a day.

Vegetarian Omega-3 Oil Sources

Although there are omega-3 oils in most green leafy vegetables, the amounts are generally insignificant. Purslane, a green leafy vegetable rarely used in salads any longer, is an excellent source of omega-3 oil, however.

Adding flaxseed oil or using flaxseed meal in baking can add a great deal of omega-3 oil to your diet. Flaxseed oil is 52 percent omega-3 oil that your body metabolizes to a more active form. Hence, because there is a little metabolism involved, it is not quite as good as fish oil.

Flaxseed oil is sold in health food stores and even some supermarkets as bottled oil, or in capsules as a supplement. The simplest way to get omega-3 oil daily is to put a tablespoon of flaxseed oil on

---

Table 12.2

Polyunsaturated Fat Content of Commonly Available Fish

Fish	Omega-3 Oil, grams per 3.5 ounce serving*
Tuna, canned in water	0.8–3.0
Herring	1.6–3.1
Mackerel	1.1–3.0
Salmon	1.4–3.0
Snapper	0.5–0.7
Rainbow trout	0.6–1.4
Flounder	0.5–1.1

*Variation is due to season, water temperature, and the food the fish have been eating. The colder the water, the higher the omega-3 oil content.

your high-fiber cereal each day along with your soy milk. Each time you do that simple procedure, you are taking two steps toward a longer life free from prostate cancer.

Cooking with Oils

You can purchase high-omega-3 cooking oils, mayonnaise, and a spread that tastes like butter. Following are some recommendations for cooking with these oils:

Frying and deep-fat cooking. Select oils that work at high heat. These include peanut, high-oleic sunflower, and high-oleic safflower oils.

Baking and sautéing. Select medium-heat oils, which include canola, soy, and walnut oils.

Light sautéing and sauces. Medium-heat oils are necessary. The champion is olive oil, followed by high-oleic sunflower, walnut, soy, and pumpkin seed oils.

Oils for soups and salads. You can directly add flaxseed oil as a fortifier and use olive oil for everything else. When out of olive oil, use canola oil.

Mayonnaise. Use low-fat canola oil mayonnaise and canola oil spread.

Learn to use olive oil on crusty breads as a spread or dip. Once you become accustomed to this, you'll wonder how you ever did it any other way.

FISH OIL SUPPLEMENTS

I recommend a diet rich in fish. Not everyone likes fish, some don't eat enough, and others simply can't eat it for a variety of reasons. The fish oil supplements available in most supermarkets, drug, and health food stores are excellent and they have been proven effective.

These supplements are sold as fish oil supplements, and in some cases as EPA, which stands for eicosapentaenoic acid, the most important of the omega-3 oils.

However you use them, two capsules daily can go a long way to improve your health and prevent cancer.

13

Protect Prostate Health with Herbs

We are living through an herbal renaissance that has people using all sorts of plant derivatives to cure or prevent every health problem known. Indeed, many modern pharmaceutical preparations have their roots in herbal remedies.

Prostate problems, particularly enlargement of the prostate or benign hypertrophy of the prostate (BHP), have proven to be responsive to herbal remedies. When a man's prostate grows inward in BHP, urinary problems start to occur. For instance, as his bladder gets full, he goes to urinate, the flow is very slow, emptying is incomplete, and he needs to urinate frequently.

Any man who has any or all of the BHP symptoms listed should see his physician who, if examination warrants, will probably refer him to a urologist. (Do not try to self-diagnose, because these same symptoms can also indicate far more serious problems.)

There are a number of herbal remedies recommended for this problem; saw palmetto, for instance, works quite well. It is not known whether any herbal remedy can prevent prostate cancer, but supporting prostate health is a vital part of prevention. An herbal remedy may be able to help you do just that.

Benign Prostatic Hypertrophy Symptoms

- Urgency/Inability. The need to urinate accompanied by an inability to urinate satisfactorily.
- Initiation. In spite of a full bladder, the inability to produce a urine stream, possibly only achieving a dribble.
- Frequent nocturnal urgency. The need to urinate at night.
- Unsatisfied voiding. The feeling you need to go again right after urination.
- Blood in the urine. This is rare with simple BHP.
- Urinary tract infections.

SAW PALMETTO

Over eight well-designed clinical studies have proven that saw palmetto, the sabal palm, is effective against BHP. Indeed, in double-blind studies, its performance was equal to the two most popular prescription drugs, and in one, it scored better. Quantitative analysis in which prostate gland size is evaluated by ultrasonic techniques proved it shrinks the prostate.

Saw palmetto grows wild in the southeastern United States and is found in other subtropical areas of the world. Tea made from its dark berries became an herbal remedy for urinary problems so long ago that its origin is lost in time. In the nineteenth century, the extract of saw palmetto berries was used as a treatment for prostate enlargement. It works well, but rather than attempt to make tea from the berries, it is better to use a commercial extract prepared by experts because saw palmetto's active chemical components are soluble in alcohol and other solvents.

Saw palmetto berries contain plant materials that modify estrogen receptors. In doing this, they also slow the conversion of testosterone to dihydrotestosterone (DHT), the compound that causes the prostate to keep on growing after middle age. Saw palmetto's components also compete with testosterone and DHT uptake by prostate gland cells. Besides the ingredient that slows DHT production, saw palmetto contains some flavonoids that bear a resemblance to those found in soy (see chapter 4).

Saw palmetto also has anti-inflammatory properties. This could explain why some men who had a high PSA test show a normal PSA reading after using saw palmetto. If the test was originally elevated as a result of an inflamed prostate, the anti-inflammatory effect could explain the results quite nicely.

If you don't have BHP, but your family history shows an above-average risk of prostate cancer, you might possibly reduce your risk by taking saw palmetto. After all, it reduces DHT production, which increases prostate cancer risk. Genetic counseling (discussed in chapter 1) can help you make a decision if done in concert with a urologist.

Early stages of BHP require about 300 to 350 milligrams of saw palmetto extract daily. In those cases where it is effective, results begin to show in about four weeks, and by six weeks they should be obvious. For a person taking saw palmetto as a preventive, the dose for mild BHP would be appropriate.

Contraindications

Saw palmetto could conceivably mask an above-average PSA test and therefore prevent early cancer detection. So, if you are using saw palmetto, make sure you discuss it with your physician when he is evaluating your PSA test.

If you have been taking a prescription drug for BHP and want to try saw palmetto, discuss and plan out your transition with a physician. Saw palmetto provides physiologically active chemicals just like any prescription drug, and shifting from one medication to another should be done carefully and cautiously. Work with your physician; don't take chances.

STINGING NETTLE

Although this herb enjoys a reputation for helping men through urinary and possibly prostate problems, there is no evidence regarding its use in prostate cancer prevention. Therefore, there is nothing I can contribute about its use. Its name is sure to emerge, however, if you consult a book on herbs or an herbalist. Be sure to ask for clinical proof of any claims made.

14

Drink Tea

If you use a caffeinated beverage, commit yourself to cancer prevention and choose tea instead of coffee or caffeinated sodas. Green tea is better than black tea, but drinking either tea is better than other beverage choices. Such a switch will reduce cancer risk.

Green tea is made from tea leaves that are picked and remain unprocessed. These tea leaves are rich with antioxidants and have proven to reduce cancer risk very effectively. Indeed, heavy smokers who drink green tea have about half the lung cancer rate of smokers who don't drink green tea.

Black tea is made from the same leaves, but after harvest, the leaves go through a fermentation process. This imparts both the dark color and the distinctively rich flavor. It also explains why the tea is black. This process also makes the caffeine more readily available.

A cup of black tea contains from 35 to 50 milligrams of caffeine; however, it's usually closer to 35 milligrams. Brewed and instant coffees generally provide from 100 to 150 milligrams of caffeine, with 125 milligrams being a reasonable average. So, if you currently start your day with a cup of coffee, you could take three cups of tea to get the came caffeine boost. Green tea contains even less caffeine, so you could probably take four cups. Green tea is also available decaffeinated if you wish to avoid caffeine's effects.

Although scientific studies indicate that tea drinkers have less cancer, the research doesn't identify what's at work. It could be the tannins found in tea. These materials are really part of a large class of materials scientifically called lignins. Studies have shown that lignins are effective antioxidants and they do reduce cancer risk.

Recent research has proven that as people age, tea drinkers have better bone density—or bone strength—than those who don't drink tea. This supports the observations that indicate the lignins have a positive effect on the processes that maintain a strong bone matrix. These same processes have a role in cancer prevention.

Tea with milk has a modest advantage over tea taken black. The milk protein modestly bonds some of the tannins in tea, which have an astringent effect. Tannins cause a degree of bitterness and can be irritating to some people's mouths.

15

Exercise

Men who exercise regularly (at least four hours weekly) and maintain good fitness have about half the prostate cancer risk of men who don't exercise. Other studies have consistently proven regular exercise also reduces colorectal cancer risk in both men and women. Maintaining an exercise program (and keeping fit, as discussed in the next chapter) is probably the simplest thing a man can do to reduce his risk.

When you exercise vigorously, do you feel hot? Do you sweat? Do you notice that your heart beats faster? During exercise your body core temperature increases by 1 or 2 degrees, depending on how aggressively you exercise. Two degrees doesn't seem like much, but it translates to a 35 percent metabolic rate increase! That's a lot. Perspiring is your body's way of cooling itself, because evaporating sweat takes away heat. An increased pulse rate means your heart is pumping faster to get blood, more specifically, oxygen, to the muscles and removing wastes, mostly carbon dioxide.

If you monitored your levels of by-products of testosterone metabolism before and after exercise, you'd notice a slight but measurable decrease due to the increase in metabolism. If you compared testosterone levels in one hundred men who exercise regularly to one hundred men who don't exercise, you'd notice the exercisers have a slightly but consistently lower level. This means a lower prostate cancer risk.

Remember, we're specifically discussing vigorous exercise during which you perspire—that is, aerobic rather than anaerobic exercise. *Aerobic* means "with air"; *anaerobic* means "without air." Aerobic exercise works the large muscle groups, such as the arms and legs, and also involves other muscle groups in the abdomen and back. You still breathe during anaerobic exercise, such as weight lifting, but unless you pump the weights up and down rapidly for a long time, you don't raise your pulse rate enough to elevate your metabolism significantly.

Aerobic exercise challenges your cardiovascular system to supply sufficient oxygen to make energy for your muscles. Your heart rises to the occasion by increasing its rate—you then breathe more rapidly and deeply to get the necessary oxygen to your muscles.

Aerobic exercise, such as running, brisk walking, and cycling, will elevate metabolism when performed for a sustained period, say, twenty to sixty minutes. This is called a "training effect" because it trains your cardiovascular system to meet the increased demands and build muscles. Jogging requires a minimum of fifteen minutes, while a brisk walk should be done for at least twenty-five minutes. These times are determined by how long it takes your heart to reach and maintain a training rate; a sampling is given in Table 15.1.

A good contrast to a twenty- or thirty-minute jog is to run a 100-yard (or meter) dash. You finish in less than twenty to thirty seconds but find yourself gasping for air for about three minutes at the finish line. The reason you gasp is that your muscles produced the energy for the dash by using energy reserves that don't require air. This creates an energy debt that must be repaid and it calls for oxygen to regenerate the high-energy reserves—this leaves you gasping.

An analogy in everyday life would be running to catch a bus, or running up stairs quickly. The gasping for breath afterward is simply your body demanding repayment of the oxygen debt you cre-

Table 15.1

Aerobic Exercise Programs

30 Minutes	50 Minutes
Jogging, road or machine	Brisk walk
Cross-country skiing, snow or machine	Sensible bicycling or
Rowing, on water or machine	stationary cycling
Aerobic stepping or dancing	In-line skating
Mini-trampoline	Swimming
Stair stepping	

ated. Your body can handle these anaerobic oxygen-debt incidents better if you exercise aerobically on a regular basis. Aerobic exercise builds better all-around capacity, even for anaerobic exercise.

WHAT'S THE BEST EXERCISE FOR YOU?

The best exercises for you are the ones you will do regularly. Be sure to vary your regular exercise routine and work different muscle groups. For example, jog and cycle when the weather is nice and use an indoor rowing machine or cycle, for example, when it is inclement.

A good active sport also helps to keep you fit. You simply need to use some common sense. Brisk sets of tennis with active opponents are good exercise. Consider racquetball, volleyball, downhill skiing, soccer, basketball, and other sports that increase your pulse for over thirty minutes and leave you perspiring.

Obviously there are many exercise methods, so there is something for everyone; no excuses! Don't use motorized devices, with the exception of treadmills, as they don't have the same training effect because your energy output is reduced by the motor. In contrast, the treadmill works because it's just the road that's moving; you're simply keeping up.

Working with weights, or anaerobic exercise, also has a very important place in total body fitness. Sensible weight workouts convert body fat to muscle. Muscle has a higher metabolic rate and contributes to body fitness. The best way to pursue a weight program is at a fitness center, with a knowledgeable trainer.

I have worked with many people in my career and without exception, I have learned that everyone can exercise. Of course, if you have a chronic illness such as arthritis or asthma, you will have to search for an exercise that works for you, but a little investigation and asking an expert will put you on the road to fitness. People who don't exercise generally excuse themselves by not finding time. I personally found that the only way I could find time to exercise regularly was to get up an hour earlier every day. Statistics prove that people who decide to exercise after work are more likely to quit than people who exercise before work; you may want to give this strategy a try yourself.

16

Maintain Fitness

Men who maintain good fitness levels have a much lower risk of prostate cancer. Virtually every study conducted confirms that being fit pays big health dividends. The bad news, however, is that most people don't know how fitness is measured.

Weight and height charts found in schools, your doctor's office, in newspapers, on scales, and elsewhere give ideal weight and height based on longevity. Those ideals don't have anything to do with fitness, however; they're about weight. Fitness is about body fat. A man's weight for his age and height can easily be, and often is, just fine, but he can be very unfit as determined by what percentage of his body weight is fat.

BODY COMPOSITION

Your body is divided into two parts: lean body mass (LBM) and fat. LBM has a high metabolic rate and fat has a very low—almost non-existent—metabolic rate. Fat is nature's insulator and is relatively inert. People with high LBM generally have a higher metabolism. It follows that their bodies metabolize unwanted materials more rapidly and eliminate them. The more fat you have, the greater is your ability to store unwanted by-products of metabolism, environmental toxins, and other wastes.

Whenever scientists search for environmental toxins in human bodies, they study body fat. Because it is inert tissue, unwanted toxins can remain there undisturbed. Indeed, there have been cases in which men who lost lots of weight developed unusual illnesses that were traced to toxic materials that had been stored in their body fat.

Ideally, you should be about 13 percent body fat, but you are healthy at 15 percent. Once you reach 18 percent body fat, you're too fat. In contrast, an athlete in good shape might come in at about 10 percent, and some runners even less than that. Try to maintain 13 percent body fat!

Nonrunning athletes, such as discus or shot put throwers, with about 10 percent body fat usually will be classified on the height/weight charts as "overweight," and on some charts as "obese" (20 percent over ideal) because their LBM is much higher, dense, and weighs more than fat. That's why we discuss body composition instead of weight when we talk about fitness.

Because fat floats, your LBM is your weight in water. This weight compared to land weight will yield LBM. Take the following example:

Height	6 feet
Weight on land	200 pounds
Weight under water	174 pounds
Weight of fat	26 pounds
Percent of fat	26/200 = 13 percent

According to a height/weight chart, a 200-pound, 6-foot man should weigh 179 to 185 pounds. In the case given above, however, this man's body composition indicates that he's fit.

DETERMINING YOUR BODY FAT PERCENTAGE

Weighing oneself in water is obviously difficult. You can now purchase a kit to measure your body fat; it consists of a caliper you use to pinch yourself in various places. That, coupled with weight, height, waist, and wrist measurements, gives a pretty good body fat estimate. There are also scales that do it by measuring body density with sound waves.

If you have access to a swimming pool or a pool that is about 4 feet deep, you can estimate your body fat by how well you float. Either curl into a ball or lay on your back, blow all the air from your lungs, and see what happens.

- 25 percent body fat: You float!
- 22 percent body fat: You will just barely float.
- 20 percent body fat: You can't stay afloat unless you move your arms and legs.
- 15 percent body fat: You will slowly sink, even if you have air in your lungs.
- 13 percent body fat: You will sink even with air in your lungs.

You should strive for a body composition that lets you sink slowly when you exhale.

INCREASING LBM

Increasing your LBM calls for exercise that convers some body fat to muscle (see chapter 15). In the process, you'll also build more bone density and increase strength in tendons and connective tissues, especially if you follow the diet plan in chapter 3. The best approach is to combine some sensible dieting with exercise to achieve your objective more quickly and effectively. We'll look at sensible ways to diet in the next chapter.

17

Monitor Your Caloric Intake

As we discussed in the last chapter, people with lower body fat always have a lower cancer risk. Becoming fit involves a combination of exercise (see chapter 15) and sensible weight loss. In order to lose weight sensibly, you should understand the basics of calorie balance. There are too many diet books, commercial weight-loss programs, weight-loss clinics, herbs, nostrums, and experts to count, so it's important to know the truth about dieting.

The relationship between calories and weight loss is simple: If you burn more calories than you consume as food, you'll lose weight. If you consume more calories as food, you'll gain weight. So how is it that some diets claim that you can eat all you want and still lose weight?

In 1847, a diet was published in which you were allowed to eat all the meat, fish, fat, and whiskey you wanted. The only other food allowed was one potato. You could substitute for the potato an apple, a serving of corn, or a few other vegetables. The trick to this diet was that it limited carbohydrates to about 60 grams daily.

Since then, this diet has reappeared in many shapes and forms. It works on a very simple principle: You need about 60 grams of carbohydrate daily to maintain an important metabolic function called the *citric acid cycle*. When you follow the low-carbohydrate dietary strategy, all your energy will come from your protein and fat.

Because the citric acid cycle is barely functioning under the limiting conditions of such diets, all fat is only partially metabolized and protein is, at best, a poor energy source and is wasted. You can keep up this diet indefinitely if you can stand it, and you will keep losing weight until you reach some level of weight equilibrium. Then what will happen? When you go off such a diet, you'll gain weight rapidly for the same reason you lost weight rapidly. Your body will immediately rebuild its carbohydrate (glycogen) reserves. Each pound of glycogen (animal starch) requires 3 or 4 pounds of water. So, if you restore 1 pound of glycogen, you gain 4 to 5 pounds.

Many experts say this way of dieting is unwise, if not downright dangerous to your health, for several of the following reasons:

- It elevates the factors that cause heart disease.
- It eliminates all the cancer-preventing factors in fruits and vegetables.
- It includes, indeed, encourages all the factors found in high-protein, high-fat foods that increase the risk of many cancers, not just prostate.
- It eliminates all the factors that prevent the diseases of aging, which include bowel troubles, cataracts, Alzheimer's disease, bone loss, and others.

CALORIES AND BASAL METABOLIC RATE

About two-thirds of our daily calories go to basal metabolism—the energy required just to keep our bodies alive. Even while you're sleeping, your heart still beats, your temperature remains at 98.6 degrees, your kidneys continue to produce urine, and so on. These functions, and myriad others, go on twenty-four hours a day. To calculate your approximate basal metabolic rate, do the following:

- Determine your height in inches.
- Subtract 60.
- Multiply by 110.
- Add 110.

For example, for a 6-foot-tall man, the calculations would look like this:

72 inches – 60 inches = 12 inches
12 x 110 = 1,320
1,320 + 110 = 1,430 calories daily

These results can vary with a number of factors:

Body fat. Body fat insulates so you don't need as many calories to maintain body temperature.

Environmental temperature. Low environmental temperature means more calories are devoted to maintaining temperature. High environmental temperature means more calories are devoted to cooling the body.

Overall physical condition. Good condition requires a low heart rate; poor condition requires a higher heart rate.

Table 17.1 illustrates the metabolic rates of a number of different men as determined by body height, weight, and age. You'll notice that the basal metabolic rate (BMR) declines with age. The three weights given for each height are ideal, overweight, and obese.

You can approximate the number of calories you consume above your BMR in daily activities by using some convenient formulas.

Daily Physical Activity

Sedentary person (sits most of the time)	0.2 BMR
Moderately active person (salesperson, teacher)	0.3 BMR
Active person (worker on feet all day)	0.4 BMR

Table 17.1

Metabolic Rate/Calories per Twenty-Four Hours

Height	Weight	Age					
		20	30	40	50	60	70
5' 10"	160	1,819	1,715	1,660	1,632	1,573	1,491
	180	1,915	1,805	1,747	1,718	1,656	1,570
	200	2,011	1,895	1,835	1,804	1,739	1,648
6' 0"	170	1,896	1,787	1,730	1,701	1,639	1,554
	190	1,992	1,877	1,817	1,787	1,722	1,632
	210	2,088	1,967	1,904	1,873	1,805	1,711
6' 2"	180	1,992	1,877	1,817	1,787	1,722	1,632
	200	2,088	1,967	1,904	1,873	1,805	1,711
	210	2,145	2,021	1,957	1,925	1,855	1,758

Vigorous exercise

0.055 cal/pound (per minute)

Fast jog (about 7 minutes/mile)
Swimming (vigorously)
Nordic Track or rowing machine (higher level)
Road cycling (brisk >13 MPH)

Moderate exercise

0.04 cal/pound (per minute)

Moderate jogging (8 minutes/mile)
Swimming (slow but consistent)
Road cycling (<13 MPH)
Nordic Track or rowing machine (lower level)

Using this information, you can develop a daily caloric table. Let's look at an example.

190-Pound Man, Age 40
BMR: 1,817 calories/24 hours
Daily activity (0.3 X 1,817) = 545 calories
Exercise: 30 minutes moderate (190 X 0.04 X 30) = 228
Total daily calories: 2,590 calories (low, 2,350; high, 2,650)

If the man in our above example, wants to take off the extra 10 pounds he's carrying that increase his prostate cancer risk, he's got to establish a total caloric deficit of 33,000 calories (10 pounds at 3,300 calories per pound). His average daily caloric expenditure is about 2,600 calories.

Suppose he cuts out 1,000 calories daily, down to 1,600 calories:

33,000 calories (10 pounds) ÷ 1,000 =
33 days spent at about 1,600 calories.

SOME TIPS ON CUTTING BACK

In general, fad diets don't work. On the other hand, self-discipline works very well. If you cut out one 300-calorie dessert daily, eat one meal of only a salad consisting of lettuce, tomatoes, some broccoli, and carrots, with no salad dressing, drink no alcoholic beverages, and increase your exercise by 50 percent, you will achieve the goal much faster. You will convert more fat to LBM and still maintain the caloric deficit. You can also follow some simple advice.

- Eat for bulk. An apple has about 150 calories (so does a square of chocolate or a dollop of butter). Eat the apple, and stop using butter, candy, and sweets.
- Snack on carrots. Supermarkets sell small, cleaned carrots in plastic bags. Take a bag with you daily. When you need a snack, start munching on carrots.

- Drink or take a fiber supplement twenty to thirty minutes before each meal (see chapter 7). It will make you feel full and you'll be able to eat less.
- Whenever people you're with are drinking alcoholic beverages, have a glass of club soda instead.

18

Take a Multiple Vitamin and Mineral Supplement Daily

In order to function normally, your body requires nineteen vitamins and minerals daily in addition to protein, fat, carbohydrates, and fiber. These requirements are expressed in terms of the recommended daily intake (RDI). Vitamins and most minerals are required in very small (trace) quantities. For example, every day you need just 400 micrograms (400 millionths of a gram) of the B vitamin folic acid. In contrast, the calcium requirement is comparatively large, ranging from 1,000 milligrams (1 gram) for most women up to about age fifty to 1,200 milligrams after that age. Magnesium's requirement is somewhat midway; you need 200 to 400 milligrams (0.4 gram) daily. With the exception of calcium and magnesium, all your vitamin and mineral needs can be packed into a single large tablet. Don't leave anything to chance; ensure your nutrition by adding supplements to avoid any possible marginal deficiencies.

While there is no direct scientific evidence that taking a daily multiple vitamin and mineral supplement will prevent prostate cancer, a number of benefits are worth considering: Niacin, a B vitamin, works at the DNA level in the cell nucleus with an enzyme that repairs DNA. Being sure you have sufficient niacin makes sense. Similarly, folic acid, another B vitamin, is essential in DNA synthesis and in the way in which genes are expressed. Data has accumulated that indicates folic acid shortfalls predispose people to cancer. It makes sense to be sure your folic acid is up to optimum levels.

Supplement your diet with at least 50 percent of the RDI for all nineteen vitamins and minerals. Why this amount? The diet plan and advice in this book will supply the RDI for most of the required nutrients; however, because our major dietary objective is reducing prostate cancer risk, a little variety could be lost, and some nutrients—primarily iron, magnesium, and calcium—will fall a little short. Supplementation is an easy way of insuring that all nutrients are present in adequate supply, any excess will be additional insurance.

I recommend a daily supplement that provides the vitamins and minerals in the amounts listed in Table 18.1. It is important that your supplement contains all these vitamins within 20 percent of the values shown here.

Few products precisely satisfy all these criteria. Usually the product you select will have less calcium and magnesium. If this is true, don't worry; you should probably take extra calcium anyway. Your diet already contains excess phosphorus and about 20 percent of the magnesium you need, so if the product you select comes to within 20 percent of the calcium, magnesium, and phosphorus listed in Table 18.1, it's fine. Don't select a supplement that varies by more than that amount.

COMMON QUESTIONS ABOUT SUPPLEMENT USE

Question: Aren't excess vitamins and minerals just excreted, making expensive urine?

Answer: Even if you're starving, your body will lose some vitamins and minerals daily through excretion. Under those conditions, your

Table 18.1

Basic Supplement

Nutrient Vitamin	Amount per Tablet*	Percent U.S. RDI
Vitamin A (as beta-carotene)	2,500 I.U.** (500 mcg RE***)	50
Vitamin D	200 I.U. (5 mcg)	50
Vitamin E	15 I.U. (5 mg alpha-tocopherol equivalents)	50
Vitamin C	30 mg	50
Folic acid	0.2 mg	50
Thiamin (B_1)	0.75 mg	50
Riboflavin (B_2)	0.86 mg	50
Niacin	10 mg	50
Vitamin B_6	1 mg	50
Vitamin B_{12}	3 mcg	50
Biotin	0.15 mg (150 mcg)	50
Pantothenic acid	5 mg	50

Nutrient Minerals

Calcium	125 mg	25
Phosphorus	180 mg	40
Iodine	75 mcg	50
Iron	9 mg	50
Magnesium	50 mg	12.5
Copper	1 mg	50
Zinc	1 mg	50
Selenium	50 mcg	****
Manganese	0.5 mg	****
Chromium	50 mcg	****
Molybdenum	30 mcg	****

* Two tablets provide 100 percent U.S. RDI for all nutrients except calcium, phosphorus, and magnesium, as explained on page 88.
** International Units.
*** Microgram retinol equivalents.
**** U.S. RDI not established.

urine is truly expensive. If your blood levels of nutrients are high, your urine levels will also be higher; that's normal human physiology.

Question: What's the upper limit of safety for vitamins and minerals?

Answer: Up to about ten times the RDI of vitamins and minerals is safe for normal people. Some are safe at many times that level.

Question: Isn't it expensive to take vitamins and minerals?

Answer: Our society spends about $1.00 per capita daily on soft drinks. Is that expensive? The average adult woman spends $1.00 daily on her hair. Is that expensive? Expensive is only meaningful by comparison. The recommended multiple vitamin and mineral supplements and the other vitamins, fiber, and omega-3 oils discussed are less than 75 cents daily. Only you can decide if your health is worth that much.

19

Drink Alcohol
Only in Moderation

Epidemiologists have determined that alcohol is a risk factor in cancer. Cancer research regarding alcohol has created a dilemma, however. Heart disease is unequivocally the greatest killer of both men and women and moderate alcohol consumption clearly reduces heart disease risk. (Thanks to its antioxidant content, red wine has a *slight* edge over other alcohol sources in reducing heart disease.) At the same time, alcohol also increases the risk of all cancers, prostate cancer included. So what do you do?

Analyze your personal relationship with alcohol. If you have a glass of wine with dinner, enjoy a beer after an afternoon working in the yard, or relax with a cocktail before dinner with your significant other, you're helping avoid heart disease and definitely not increasing your cancer risk—especially if you take the steps outlined in the rest of this book.

At the high end of alcohol use, about three or four drinks daily, your risk of cancer is 41 percent higher than someone who doesn't drink alcohol at all but otherwise is exactly like you. That's a clear conclusion. Besides, if you're having over three alcoholic drinks daily, you're not drinking in moderation. Bad habits tend to come in clusters, so if you're having three drinks daily, you likely have some other bad habits; for example, you don't exercise, you don't eat three to five vegetables daily, or you eat more than 4 ounces of red meat daily. If you average only a glass of wine, a beer, or a cocktail daily, you don't incur a statistically significant risk.

A man asked me once if he could save his drinks up for a week and have a "blast" every Saturday night. Epidemiological studies can't differentiate between taking seven glasses of wine, seven beers, or seven cocktails one night a week, and having one drink each night over the course of a week. Common sense tells us, however, that you shouldn't drink that way. Your body would pay a high price if you did.

Alcohol is actually a deadly toxin, because at certain levels it can affect brain function. At high enough levels, it can cause the brain to stop functioning entirely. That's why alcohol is rapidly metabolized; your liver has an enzyme system to metabolize alcohol into carbon dioxide and water while extracting its energy.

An average 150-pound person can metabolize the equivalent of about one alcoholic beverage an hour. So, if you're average and at a party, you might have three drinks in an evening of, say, two to two and a half hours, and by the time you've said your good-byes, the alcohol you consumed has been metabolized to carbon dioxide and water. Use a little common sense when drinking because your weight also tells you when to quit. If you're 120 pounds, then you should nurse the drinks along and just have two during the party.

I recommend, however, that you stick to no more than one drink a day; if you have two in one evening, abstain the following day. Alcohol's effects on your system are not fully understood. Sophisticated biochemical studies are uncovering a complex involvement of an insulin factor, a vitamin-D metabolite, and alcohol.

There are other health concerns to consider as well. While your liver is handling the alcohol, other things like fat and sugar line up for their turns. If you drink more than the liver can handle in a reasonable time, fat starts accumulating in the liver and sugar builds up in the blood. Your triglycerides and blood fats also become elevated.

Alcohol also produces free radicals as it is metabolized, and its mere presence causes a modest decline in antioxidants, especially vitamins C and E. Both of these effects increase cancer risk. Some research suggests that repeated heavy alcohol use increases hormone output. That probably explains why heavy drinking causes above-average breast and prostate cancer risk.

Another side of alcohol is its ability to dehydrate. In fact, the bad effects from too much alcohol—a hangover —are usually the result of dehydration and elevated blood sugar. So, be sure to drink lots of water. A good rule to follow is to have one full 8-ounce glass of water for each drink during the evening. This helps restore fluid loss and will keep you healthy. You can offset the alcohol even more by substituting a glass of orange juice for one glass of water. Orange juice, in addition to being an antioxidant powerhouse, is also the best, most practical potassium source available. Potassium is indirectly depleted by alcohol.

A PRACTICAL APPROACH

Learn to drink moderately, and keep the "one drink daily" rule in mind. A nice wine can make a good meal a dining experience. With a little common sense, you can enjoy it and not worry about any consequences for your health. There are none, if you use caution.

20

Don't Play
Environmental Roulette

Prostate cancer, similar to every other cancer, can be initiated by environmental factors. Our environment is generally safe; in ancient Rome, a seemingly pristine time, only 50 percent of people made it to age twenty. Now, over 50 percent of people live to about age sixty; before long, that average will reach age eighty. That means, however, that we will have more exposure to all sorts of chemicals. Indeed, about 1,500 new chemicals are introduced annually. Although about half are tested for safety, we haven't the foggiest idea of how they will interact with the 1,500 from the year before or the other 750 that aren't tested, let alone those introduced ten years previously. Common sense dictates caution and self-protection.

Numerous studies have been conducted that look at cancer rates among people who work in the chemical industry. The best studies compare people who work with and around the chemicals to those who work far from the chemicals; for example, accountants in the home office and workers in the plant. These studies, undertaken worldwide over many decades among many companies and industries, and with a wide variety of chemicals, lead to one conclusion:

The more you are exposed to chemicals, especially solvents and fuels, the more likely you are to develop cancer.

Pesticides are another environmental factor of which to be aware. Pesticides are generally built around hormones that will affect either the male or female of the species. The data showing they can cause cancer, especially breast cancer, is so strong that the dean of a well-known Ivy League medical school has declared that they are carcinogenic.

WHAT YOU CAN DO

Take some commonsense precautions, such as the following:

- Wash your fruits and vegetables. A small amount of dishwashing liquid in cold water works fine. Let them soak a few minutes, swishing them around, then rinse.
- Use appropriate precautions when handling solvents and chemicals, such as gloves, masks, and other appropriate clothing.
- Wash your hands and areas exposed to solvents, garden chemicals, automotive fuels, and other materials.
- Don't breathe fumes! Get away from them! Open windows!
- Maintain appropriate citizenship with respect to local water and air pollution. Be responsible when using and disposing of household chemicals, and do everything you can to reduce your contribution to pollution.

Conclusion

After writing this book and reflecting on all the information it contains, I am struck by the simplicity and wide-reaching power of the approach to prostate cancer prevention in this book. It's simple because it calls for establishing some dietary and lifestyle habits that are not difficult by any measure, and wide reaching because these habits help prevent all cancers, heart disease, and the diseases of aging, such as cataracts. So, if the entire family adopts these habits, everyone becomes a winner and gains the prospect of living longer and living better. It is worth reviewing the basic elements of the plan one more time.

DIETARY HABITS

Eat for bulk, using fruits, vegetables, cereals, and grains. Every day, include at least five, and preferably seven, servings of fruits and vegetables. Include at least one dish with tomato sauce or a glass of tomato juice, have sliced tomatoes on a sandwich, and yes, it does help to use ketchup. Treat beans as a special vegetable and have at least one serving daily.

For snacking, use vegetables and fruits to increase your daily consumption. Make these healthy snacks a part of your everyday eating strategy.

Consume 30 grams of fiber each day. You know you're getting enough when you have one easy, light brown, firm bowel movement daily. This requires one serving a day of a high-fiber cereal and the use of whole-grain breads.

Eat red meat only occasionally; focus on fish, poultry, and fermented dairy products (cheese and yogurt) as protein sources.

Use supplements sensibly as part of an overall nutrition plan. Treat herbs with respect and use them carefully when appropriate.

LIFESTYLE

Achieve a reasonable weight and maintain regular exercise habits. Exercise sensibly five times weekly as both an adjunct to weight maintenance and to establish a consistent basal metabolic rate that is at the high end of normal. Exercise reduces cancer risk by itself and makes dietary steps even more effective. Use exercise to effectively dissipate the stress of today's complex living.

Take alcohol in moderation, and never use it as a stress reliever.

At least, have a biannual physical exam, and a PSA test annually when you're over the age of forty. Prevention is never 100 percent; however, early detection of prostate cancer taken together with the preventive steps in this book is 100 percent effective.

ATTITUDE

While researching for and writing this book, I interviewed many men who had prostate cancer, and many others who didn't but had fathers and brothers who did. The majority of these men, about 60 percent, were eager to gain and apply information that would reduce their own risk and that of their children. I was disappointedly surprised, however, by the large minority (30 to 35 percent) who had a fatalistic, "do-nothing" attitude. They reasoned that they were somehow destined to get prostate cancer, so they didn't bother with prevention. That fatalistic attitude baffles me because if we all had it, mankind would never have achieved the great heights we have reached, nor would we look forward to the next challenge. Think of it like this: Even if you only put the disease off one year, that is one more year your life will be cancer free, and you'll have the confidence of knowing you did all you could to prevent this grim disease. It seems like a "no-brainer" to me.

One final consideration is our individual responsibility to others. Focus on the example we each set for the people around us, especially the next generation, our children and grandchildren. Nutrition research proves over and over that children adopt their parents' eating and lifestyle habits. For example, children with the worst eating habits are usually those whose parents smoke and whose eating habits are compromised by tobacco's effect on taste and food preference. Each one of us can and should set an example not only for our children and loved ones, but also for all the young people we encounter throughout life.

Index

Page references followed by the letter "*t*" indicate tabular material